Dieting DISCARD Sucks

What to Do When Your Waistline Makes You Miserable

Joanne Kimes

author of *Pregnancy Sucks, Pregnancy Sucks for Men,* and *Dating Sucks*

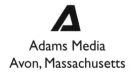

Adams Media
Avon, Massachusetts

Published by
Adams Media, an F+W Publications Company
57 Littlefield Street, Avon, MA 02322. U.S.A.
www.adamsmedia.com

ISBN 10: 1-59337-636-7
ISBN 13: 978-1-59337-636-9
Printed in the United States of America.

J I H G F E D C B A

Library of Congress Cataloging-in-Publication Data
Kimes, Joanne.
Dieting sucks / by Joanne Kimes.
    p.   cm.
ISBN 1-59337-636-7
1. Reducing diets--Popular works. 2. Weight loss--Popular works. I. Title.
RM222.2.K53 2006
    613.2'5--dc22
                        2006014730

This publication is designed to provide accurate and authoritative information with regard to the subject matter covered. It is sold with the understanding that the publisher is not engaged in rendering legal, accounting, or other professional advice. If legal advice or other expert assistance is required, the services of a competent professional person should be sought.

 —From a *Declaration of Principles* jointly adopted by a Committee of the American Bar Association and a Committee of Publishers and Associations

Many of the designations used by manufacturers and sellers to distinguish their product are claimed as trademarks. Where those designations appear in this book and Adams Media was aware of a trademark claim, the designations have been printed with initial capital letters.

This book is available at quantity discounts for bulk purchases. For information, please call 1-800-289-0963.

This book is intended as a reference volume only, not as a medical manual. The information given here is not intended as a substitute for professional fitness and medical advice. If you suspect that you have a medical problem, seek competent medical help. You should also seek your doctor's approval before you begin any diet or exercise program.

All diets identified by name within this book are the intellectual property of their respective owners and no claim of any rights thereto is being made herein. In addition, care has been taken to properly identify each of these diets by their accurate designation(s) and to utilize the trademark symbols "®" and "™" where appropriate.

The opinions presented in this book are those of the author alone and are not meant in any way to disparage the diets themselves, the trademarks associated therewith, or the diet owners. Neither the author nor the publisher is in any way associated or affiliated with the entity owning the rights to any of the diets referred to herein.

I dedicate this book to my father, Art Fink.
Thanks for a lifetime of wise words and encouragement,
and for always being there when I need you.
I love you more than you know.

contents

Chapter Three
The Real Skinny Behind Diets 49

Chapter Four
The Hell You Endure to Look Better in Jeans 83

Chapter Five
No Pain, No Gain . . . No Thank You!

Chapter Six
Motivational Tools of the Trade

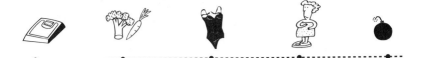

acknowledgments

A book is never written by one person alone. Well, that's not entirely true—I typed all 66,780 words of this one myself and have the jammed "S" key to prove it. But there are people who were invaluable in other ways, and I'd like to take a moment to thank them.

Thank you to my wonderful husband, Jeff, who continues to adore me despite the fact that I can no longer fit into my wedding dress. And my daughter, Emily, whom I love more than I ever thought possible. She makes me laugh every day, which is why I continue to feed her.

I'm forever grateful to my previous editor, Kate Epstein, for picking out my first submission from the slush pile years back, and turning it into the best career a stay-at-home mom could ever have. And to my new editors, Meredith O'Hayre and Jennifer Kushnier, for not only working hard on this book, but for letting me leave in some of my edgier jokes.

A big thank-you to my agent, Jeff Herman, who's guided my career as adeptly as a Seeing Eye dog.

This book was also helped by the generosity and humor of the following people, who passed on their dieting tales of woe: Hallie Rosen, AdaLynne Olifiers, Stan Zimmerman,

Mary Odson, Lisa Ritter, Carol and Mitch Metcalf, Elaine Duffy, Amy Edwards, and as always, Melissa Kimberly.

And last but not least, I'd like to thank the person who invented spell check and made it possible for none of you to ever know how atroshusly I really spell (see, I just spelled "atrociously" wrong and none of you were the wiser).

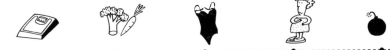

a diet book is born

Today was not a good day. I had my annual doctor's appointment and was given some really bad news. No, it wasn't a bad test result or a newfound lump. But nonetheless, the news was not good. When I stepped on that horrible doctor's scale, I was told that I had gained eleven pounds over this past year! I stared at the numbers on the scale, with the same feelings of disbelief I had when I saw Michael Jackson dangle his infant son from that infamous balcony. In both cases I was shocked at what I saw and in both cases, I felt physically sickened.

To fully understand the nature of my panic, you must understand one thing: The scale that I have at my home is one of my oldest and dearest friends. It's the first scale that I've ever owned, and it's been by my side for almost twenty years now. Whenever I step on my true blue metallic friend, it always tells me what I want to hear: I weigh less than I thought I did. Sure, on some level I know that the scale is broken. I realize that I should put it on a hard surface like the instructions say, instead of a soft carpet. And I know that I should reset the arrow to zero instead of leaving it on negative ten, where it permanently rests. But instead of doing these things, I choose to be ignorant and believe that what the scale tells me is true. I also choose to believe that blueberry scones are actually low in fat, and I don't want to be any wiser about that fact either, thank you very much.

So here I sit on my extra-wide load, having added eleven pounds to the face of the earth, and realize that I have to start yet another in a long line of diets. I must show more self-control. I must exhibit more discipline. And most of all, I must move my computer farther away from the refrigerator when I work.

The good news is that if there's one thing that I have a skill for, it's dieting (I also have a skill for saying the alphabet backwards really fast but I couldn't make much money from that, could I?). The reason that I'm so good at dieting is that I've been doing it since my early teens, when my body developed the horrible ability to develop cellulite. It was then that I discovered I could no longer get the zipper closed on my Ditto bell-bottom jeans. I went on my first diet that morning back in 1976 and went off of it around lunchtime that same day. But I learned some very important things from that experience. One, I should never start a diet on the same day they serve cinnamon rolls at school. And two, that I should have listened to my body and realized that I had the same adverse reaction to dieting as I did to my first puff of a cigarette. My body told me the diet was as toxic and unhealthy for me as that tobacco smoke was. And it was right. After each unsuccessful diet, I seemed to gain back more weight than I had lost in the first place, which set me up for a lifetime of dieting.

I know all the challenges and misery that dieters go through, and I believe that it's best not to face them alone. Why should you have to go through the agony of dieting all by your lonesome when there are so many others who are struggling with the same obstacles that you're faced with? Not only will having someone with you make the road much easier to travel, but you'll also have someone there to stop you when you're tempted to pull over at a fast-food joint along the way.

If you're contemplating starting a diet, or if you're already on one, I offer you my sincere condolences. I also offer this book filled with humor, compassion, and, I hope, very few typos. By reading it, not only will you get the support and understanding that you so desperately need, you'll also burn about 200 calories just by sitting on your ass and reading it. I don't promise to make you lose 30 pounds in thirty days, nor do I guarantee that you'll have less body fat or an ass as hard as day-old bread. What I do promise is a book that contains lots of dieting wisdom, dieting tips, and not even one itty-bitty carbohydrate.

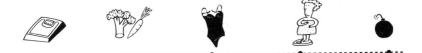

chapter one

the last straw . . . berry shake!

D-I-E-T. There's no doubt about it. It's a four-letter word. Just typing that combination of letters in that specific order fills me with horror, despair, and severe hunger pains. Diets have plagued millions of people ever since the invention of high-fructose corn syrup and desserts with creamy centers. Throughout the years, they've been responsible for more irritability and headaches than automated phone operators and have been a hardship for everyone to endure, except of course for the companies that manufacture sugar substitutes.

Nevertheless, diets are as much a part of today's lifestyle as teeth whiteners and penile enhancement pop-up ads. That's because throughout history, there have never been more overweight people and more ways to become overweight. If you're heavy, it may be because you're a late-night snacker or a fast-food junkie. Or maybe you're an all-day grazer or someone who considers a supersized meal to be

1

merely an appetizer. As you can see, there are many ways to become overweight, and all of the roads are happy ones paved with fresh baked goods and all-you-can-eat buffets.

I myself am heavy and have been a dieter for more than twenty years. I grew up in Los Angeles, which is the land of the emaciated figure. Here, the ideal body weight for a woman is a few pounds shy of organ failure. To make matters worse, I come from a family that is extremely weight-conscious. My mother, for instance, stands about five feet tall and weighs in at only 95 pounds. She's a very disciplined woman and is the only person in history who can indeed eat but one Lay's potato chip. My sister is built the same way and weighed less than I do when she was nine months pregnant. Yes, I am indeed the fat one in the family. The big, blubberous, black sheep of the family whose biggest fantasy is to be told that I was adopted just so I could make sense of this horrible injustice.

How heavy am I, you may ask? I'd be happy to share my weight with you, but it fluctuates more than the Dow Jones Averages. At this moment, I'd estimate that I'm carrying around an extra 25 pounds. If you think about it, that's like strapping a toddler to my ass and inner thighs. My personal path to poundage is that I'm quite a big eater. I'm very much like a goldfish, which will eat and eat until it dies. Because of this, I'm also a dieter.

If you're a dieter too, then you know the road that you traveled to get here. But just as there are many different ways to become overweight, there are many different motivating factors that make you want to start a diet. Here are some of the most popular ones.

I Don't Have Anything to Wear . . . That Fits

There are some women who put themselves together beautifully in the morning. Their wardrobe is like one big Gar-
animal collection in which everything complements every
other piece beautifully. The fabrics are soft, the fit is divine,
and the clothes are so clean, you could perform surgery on
them. I envy women like this because I'm so much the opposite. Hardly anything I own matches and even if it does, it's
inevitably stained with pudding.

Maybe you can relate. After agonizing over what to wear,
you finally decide upon an outfit for the day. But suddenly
the dressing process comes to a screaming halt, or rather
you're the one who's doing the screaming, because you can't
seem to get your stupid zipper closed. Of course, you rationalize the situation by telling yourself that you just
washed those jeans (rationalization is such a wonderful thing
and the reason why we own so many pairs of shoes). Then,
you look at the mountainous pile of laundry in the corner
and realize that you haven't done a load of darks since the
Clinton administration.

My closet is riddled with stories like this. In fact, I've
learned that as I travel through the various stages of my life,
I've gained experience, wisdom, and several inches on my
waistline. Maybe you know what I'm talking about. Maybe
you too have a closet that's as overstuffed as a Shabby Chic
sofa. Your T-shirts and hangers are pushed together like New
York City subway riders. To the naive, it appears as if you
have an enormous wardrobe, but we experienced dieters know
the truth. What you have is several different-sized wardrobes

that are used to accommodate the several different body types that you've had at different points through the years.

Let me take you on a virtual tour of the wardrobes that infest my closet:

1. Remnants of clothing from my high school days, like my purple angora sweater, which is the first thing I ever bought with my own money. Yes, I know that the only chance I have of fitting into it again is if I have my internal organs removed, but I just can't seem to throw it away.

2. A handful of clothes that stem back to my college years after I gained my freshman 15, and threw in a few pounds more for extra credit.

3. Some of my early career clothes. They're professional and tailored, and were a great way to camouflage the weight that I packed on due to the long hours, the stress of corporate backstabbing, and of course, the free bagels in the lunchroom.

4. The clothes that I bought after I got married. Before I walked down the aisle I rarely cooked. But now I have to fix actual meals consisting of the four food groups that my husband grew up on, namely starch, gravy, meat, and cheese. You see, I married someone from Missouri, the "Show Me" state. I never understood what this meant before, but I've come to learn that it means "show me the way to the pharmacy to refill my high cholesterol medication."

5. My maternity wardrobe. Not long after making my husband all of those hot cross buns, I found out I had a bun in my own oven. So of course, I had to buy myself a maternity wardrobe. Even though we've decided that

the closest thing our daughter will have to a sibling is her cat, Phoebie, I still can't seem to give away my old maternity clothes. Besides, they come in handy after those Halloween and Easter candy binges and of course, after eating that big Thanksgiving dinner.

So if you're running out of room in your closet, it may be time to shed some weight as well as a few drawers of clothing. It's either that, or earn enough money to move into a home that has a walk-in closet the size of an airplane hangar.

• The Big Belle of the Ball

One of the most common reasons to shed some of that excess body poundage is an upcoming event like a high school reunion, a wedding (especially your own), a vacation where skin-revealing clothing must be worn, and of course, a party where you expect to see an old boyfriend you never got over. You circle the date of the event on your calendar and calculate just how many pounds you need to lose each week in order to look simply fabulous in your outfit (and you thought that you'd never use your high school math when you grew up). If the event is scheduled months in advance, you'll be in fine shape. Hopefully, after the calculations are complete, you'll just have to lose a pound or so a week. Not that losing a pound or so each week is such a breeze, it's just that it's much easier than if the event were to take place next week and you'd be forced to amputate a limb in order to reach your goal weight in time.

I've discovered that I have the most successful time losing weight when I feel the pressure of an upcoming event hovering over me. To give myself even more motivation, I keep the outfit that I need to squeeze into in the kitchen, right next to the value-size bag of Bugles. I also try on the outfit every once in a while to see how much higher I can get the zipper to close. That zipper is like my own DEFCON system—if I can't get it to reach the proper level, I'll destroy the world around me.

Take last month, for instance. My good friend was getting married and I was given the wretched honor of being a bridesmaid. I bought the hideous dress that she inflicted upon me despite the fact that it made me look as if I had lost my sheep and didn't know where to find them. As if the look of the dress wasn't bad enough, I couldn't get the zipper to close, so I had to lose a few pounds to fit into it.

After starving myself for a month, the wedding day arrived and I felt just like Cinderella at her ball. After all my hard work, my dress fit like a dream. I walked in with my head held high, and my zipper held higher. But does that mean I had a great time? Absolutely not! I ended up spending most of the evening alone in a corner feeling shy and uncomfortable. The truth is that no one besides me really gives a crap about how much I weigh, and I'm always shy and uncomfortable at functions no matter what the scale says.

But Cinderella and I did have a few other things in common. For one, neither of us ended up staying past midnight—she because of the deal she made with her fairy godmother, and me because I'm so old, I fall asleep before the evening news. And just like Cinderella, I too ended up being transformed back into my old self as soon as I left the party. But that had less to do with a magic spell, and more to do with the fact that I stopped off at the nearest KFC for a bucket of Popcorn Chicken.

❝Two months before my wedding I went on Atkins and lost enough weight to fit into a size four wedding dress. But once my husband fed me that yummy bite of cake, it was all over and I couldn't get carbs in me fast enough. By the time I got back from my honeymoon I was up to a size eight!**❞**

—Melissa

If you too have been invited to a special occasion that inspires you to go on a diet, just remember that as quickly as the pounds melt away, they tend to come right back after the party is over. At least they do for me. I guess the secret for permanent weight loss is to have special occasions lined up every two weeks for the rest of your life!

If you do manage to flatten out your tummy so that you look good in a form-fitting dress, don't blow it all by eating the wrong foods before you leave. Certain foods have a tendency to make your stomach blow up more than Demi Moore's on that infamous pregnant *Vanity Fair* cover. The specific foods that you should steer clear of are:

1. Foods that are high in salt, such as soy sauce, tomato juice, or anything that's been sprinkled with a salt shaker one too many times. These foods make you retain more water than SpongeBob SquarePants does.
2. Carbonated sodas. The bubbles in these drinks tend to push out your gut.
3. Foods that are high in fat, such as cheese, burgers, and frosting. These foods take longer to digest than do

fruits and lean proteins, so they stay in your belly for a longer period of time.

4. Beans, raw vegetables, and other foods that can give you gas.

5. Sweets that are made with the sugar substitute sorbitol.

If you take these precautions and still find that your stomach is bloated, try Beano before you go out. Hopefully, there'll "be no" problems.

And Baby Makes Three . . . Additional Dress Sizes

Sure, having a baby is a wonderful experience. It gives your life new meaning and brings happiness to each and every day. It also brings a constant array of poopy diapers, nipple cream, and padded toilet seat covers, but that's a matter for a different book. Not only is having a baby a life-altering experience, it also makes for a clothes-altering one, because pregnancy can add several inches to your waistline.

If you've been pregnant, your doctor no doubt recommended that you gain 25 to 35 pounds, although if you're like me, you thought it was best to err in excess. You loved being given medical permission to eat for two, but got into trouble when you assumed that this meant two sumo wrestlers. Once you gave birth to that beautiful 6-pound bundle of joy, you quickly panicked when you calculated just how much baby fat was still left on your body.

For the first few months you couldn't even deal with trying to lose the extra weight because you were up to your sleep-deprived eyeballs in breast pumps, screaming fits, and the constant barrage of visitors who were as eager to see the baby as if you'd just given birth to George Clooney. You also thought that the extra weight would just magically vanish because you believed those rumors that breastfeeding would quickly give you your figure back. What the books failed to tell you is that when you breastfeed, you still have to eat for two . . . two double D cups that is, because your body requires many additional calories in order for it to produce milk.

So the months went by and still you seemed to be sporting your maternity clothes. It hit you that Mother Nature wants you to hold on to your baby fat like you'd hold on to a gold Krugerrand. Ms. Nature is one smart cookie and wants you to have plenty of stored-up energy to feed your baby in case your food supply runs out (she made up these rules long before there was a 7-Eleven on every corner). Finally, after months and months of nursing, you decided to take Junior off the boob—a wise decision, especially since Senior was demanding ownership rights again. You managed to shed some of the weight, but enough was left on you to make people still ask if you're pregnant (please tell me that I wasn't the only one this happened to!).

You tried to lose the weight so that you could fit back into your prepregnancy jeans, but the diets just didn't seem to work. One possible explanation for this is that pregnancy can alter your metabolism. When you're pregnant, it puts a big strain on your thyroid gland (the organ that's responsible for doing things like regulating your body temperature and metabolism). If you seem to be dieting and dieting to no avail, make an appointment with your doctor to check your thyroid. If you're lucky, maybe all you'll need is a pill to cure your ill, and your weight loss problems.

Another reason that it may be hard to get back to your prepregnancy weight is because of your postdelivery high stress level. If you're someone who eats when you're stressed, having a new baby in the house will make you eat like a member of the NFL. Sure, there are some mothers who weigh less after having a baby than they did before they got knocked up, but that's because they're so busy cleaning up after their baby all day. Not me. I found that all I did was clean up after my baby's plate of uneaten food. I'd finish the untouched PB&J sandwich, chow down on the leftover mac & cheese, and cross my fingers hoping that she wouldn't finish all of her ice-cream sundae just so that I could have a treat of my own.

It also seems that bringing a new life into this world means bringing a whole lotta junk food into your cupboards. Chicken nuggets replace Lean Cuisines, and Oreo cookies replace your fat-free SnackWell's. It's as if your kitchen got an extreme makeover by the Pillsbury Doughboy!

Yes, my procreating friend, having a baby is one huge motivating factor to start up a diet. If you feel that it's time to start counting calories as well as little piggies, then good for you. Who knows? Maybe being as sleep-deprived as you are, you won't even be aware that you're going through the hell of a diet at all.

> **"Whenever I go into a clothing store, I tell the salesgirl that I just had a baby so that I don't feel so bad about all the weight I'm still carrying. It's not a lie, really. I did have a baby. It's just that my baby is going to start second grade this fall."**
>
> —Julia

Shop till You Drop in Disgust

There are several reasons why a trip to the mall can lead directly to a diet. The first of these little motivators hits you when you can't get your ass to squeeze into what you thought of as your usual pant size. Sure, the saleslady tries to console you by saying this certain line tends to run small, but you both know the truth: you have moved up a notch in your clothing size. But unlike moving up to a de-luxe apartment in the sky, there is absolutely no joy in this kind of a move up!

The second kind of shopping disaster happens when the saleslady utters the nine ugliest words in the English language: "I'm sorry, but that doesn't come in your size." She says it in a tone of pity that's usually reserved for people wearing those spongy neck braces. Of course she'll suggest a comparable item just to be kind (and because she works on commission), but by then the damage has been done. I for one feel my self-esteem plummet faster than the price of tech stocks did during the crash of '02.

But by far the biggest motivation of all is when bathing suit season rears its ugly, spandex-covered little head. Just the thought of walking into a store filled with string bikinis and short shorts makes me want to reach for a defibrillating paddle.

As any woman who has not graced the cover of *Sports Illustrated* will tell you, bathing suit shopping is worse than getting a Pap smear, a mammogram, and a bikini wax all at the same time . . . and I'm talking about a Brazilian wax that leaves you as smooth as Barbie. You'd think that bathing suit designers would be aware of women's anxieties by now and would invent a swimsuit that can camouflage all of our trouble zones. But until that day, women are forced to subject themselves to this yearly degradation. As soon as the first crocus of spring pushes its way through the thawing ground, women around the country tremble in fear. We know that any day now, we'll have to search through the racks in a desperate attempt to find something that doesn't exist: a bathing suit that we will actually look good in without the additional purchase of a matching terry-cloth bigtop tent known as a cover-up. We stroll past the adorable bikinis like the ones we wore as a preteen and head toward the far back of the store where they keep the suits so large they can double as BBQ covers.

Fortunately, I have two ways to solve these shopping dilemmas. One, go online to any label-making Web site and order your own damn clothing labels in any size that you want, and sew them into your clothes. I know that I'd wear any article of clothing no matter how hideous, as long as it came with a size-four label. And, if you order them with the names "Chanel" and "Prada" printed on them, you'll not only impress your friends, but you'll make a heck of a lot more money at future garage sales. Second, I propose that bathing suit designers team up with world-famous magicians like David Copperfield, Lance Burton, and other masters of illusion. If these geniuses can make a whole elephant disappear, they should have no problem hiding a couple of unsightly saddlebags.

Your Annual Checkup

Just as shopping can result in the beginnings of a diet, so can going to the doctor's office. For one thing, being overweight can cause serious health risks and concerns that may warrant the need to shed some unwanted pounds. Your doctor may tell you that your blood pressure is too high or that your cholesterol level is through the roof. Or he could inform you that you're at risk of developing diabetes or heart disease. But the incident that sends more patients to Weight Watchers than anything else combined is getting on the doctor's scale.

Once a year we head to our M.D.'s office for a thorough checkup. (If you don't, you should. End of lecture.) Sure, we dread the long wait, the poking and the prodding, and the humiliating paper gown that shows more skin than Paris Hilton does. But what we fear most of all is the doctor's scale. As the nurse walks us down that long sterile hallway on our way toward the enemy, we feel as if we're a prisoner on death row heading toward the electric chair. In both instances we want the walk to last forever, and in both instances we know that the result will be life-altering.

When we get there, we slip off our shoes and mentally berate ourselves for wearing our heaviest belt, our thick wool turtleneck, and our double-strength styling gel. We climb onboard and cross our fingers in hopes of a low outcome, but know the news isn't good when the nurse shakes her head, says, "tsk, tsk, tsk," and jots down our weight in our charts like an F on our permanent record.

After going through that traumatic scale experience myself, I'm here to tell you that there are five stages of dealing with being weighed that, coincidentally, are the same ones you go through when dealing with any other kind of devastating trauma:

1. Denial: When the scale finally balances, you take a look at the resulting number in disbelief. You're convinced that either there's something wrong with the

scale or that there's suddenly been an increase in the Earth's gravitational pull.

2. Anger: After you come to your senses, the anger stage sets in. You search for anything else to blame the weight gain on but yourself. Curse that Ronald McDonald for his secret sauce, and that dastardly Colonel Sanders for his eleven herbs and spices. If it weren't for those two beasts, you wouldn't be in this mess in the first place!

3. Bargaining: Once the anger dissipates, you enter this third stage in hopes of changing your present, unacceptable situation. When dealing with death, you strike a deal with God promising that, if He cures you, you'll trade in your Hummer for a hybrid. With fat, however, you plead with Ben & Jerry's to finally come up with a low-cal version of their irresistible Phish Food Ice Cream.

4. Depression: As you enter one of the final stages, it becomes quite clear that you are indeed overweight. Once your breathing steadies and the truth becomes clear, you sink into an abyss of depression that's as deep as the crust on a Chicago-style pizza. Hey wait, don't go there. That's what got you into this mess in the first place!

5. Acceptance: Okay, okay, you weigh more than you thought you did. But it's not the worst thing in the world. It's not like they stopped rerunning episodes of *Sex and the City*! It's at this point that you enter the fifth and final stage of bereavement: acceptance. From now on, until further notice, it's goodbye cottage fries and hello cottage cheese!

The Camel's Back

Another reason to start a new diet is that you've finally had enough of being overweight. You're sick of spending so much money on food and realize that you could retire from what you've spent on ice-cream sandwiches alone. You're tired of holding in gas all day, and exhausted from camouflaging your trouble zones that seemed to have doubled in size like bread dough. In addition to being tired of the physical problems of being heavy, you're tired of the emotional problems as well.

It seems that when you're heavy, you tend to feel bad about yourself and blame all your other problems on your weight. When you get passed over for that big promotion, even though you're the hardest worker and the only employee who doesn't use the company postage meter to return J.Crew packages, you tell yourself it must be because you're fat. If your boyfriend dumps you, or you husband walks out, you tell yourself that the reason he left is because you're nothing but a big, fat, gelatinous pig (hey, you said it, I didn't). Whatever bad experience you have, you blame it on the fact that you're heavy. "If only I looked better in jeans I'd have someone to love me." "If only I had an hourglass figure instead of one like a snow globe, I'd be set in my career." If only. If only. If only.

Of course, the inherent problem that stems from this warped way of thinking is that being thin doesn't necessarily translate to being happy. Oftentimes people blame other, unrelated things for aspects of their life that they're unsatisfied with. Those who are poor think they'd be happier if they were rich. Those with small chests think their lives would be better if they had more cleavage. Sure, it all sounds good on paper, but if you look at lottery winners whose families no longer speak to them, or the not-so-fulfilling life of the bosomy Marilyn Monroe, you'll realize that things aren't always what they seem. In addition, if you blame all your problems on your weight, the self-destructive behavior becomes a vicious cycle. It seems that when you fill your mind with negative thoughts, you tend to fill your stomach with Cool Ranch Doritos.

Now that the straw has broken the camel's back, you're full of motivation to get rid of some of your extra pounds. Who knows? It could happen that if you lose weight, your boyfriend will suddenly come back to you. Or that if you look better in a pinstriped suit, you'll finally get that corner office with the view. Just remember that life isn't always fair, no matter what you weigh. The only thing that's certain is that you should *definitely* be sending back your mail-order packages on the office's dime, since no one seems to be checking.

Talking Heads, and Other Body Parts

As women, we accept that our bodies will change over the years. We know that we'll get some wrinkles, that our hearing will fade, and that one day, we'll need to tuck our boobs into our underwear. Sure, we fight the aging process every step of the way, but we know that growing old is as inevitable as death, taxes, and the UPS guy knocking on the front door whenever we're taking our morning constitutional. But we do have the power to fight some changes, and one of them is how much we weigh.

We all have our own individual limits as to what the scale can say before we give Jenny Craig a call. For some, it may only be a few pounds over our usual weight. For others, it may be when they have to move that 50-pound weight block over in order to get the scale to balance. But for many of us, it's not what the scale tells us that makes us begin a diet; it's what our bodies have to say that makes all the difference. Yes, it seems that we not only have an inner voice but an outer one as well, made up of several of our individual body parts. Here is a head-to-toe breakdown of what those parts have to say.

An extra chin: I like getting something free just like everyone else, including those zillionaire celebrities who clamor over free Oscar giftbags as if they really need a third digital camera or another rhinestone cell phone or for that matter, that all-expenses-paid trip to a tropical island to relax after their hard lifestyle of daily massages and in-house chefs who will whip up a lobster roll at their beck and call. Sorry, I just felt the need to vent. Yes, I too like getting something for free, but I draw the line at a free extra chin. It's hard to ignore an extra chin when it is telling you to lose weight, because it yells at you every time you look at a photograph of yourself. It seems that whenever you say "cheese," it hollers back, "make that nonfat cheese, ya big tub!"

Your breasts: The boobs are sort of the fried pork rinds of the body because they too are made of almost all fat. Because of this, when we women pack on the pounds, those two lard-laden vessels tend to pack them on right along with us. You can hear your breasts telling you to put down that fudge sauce every time your top blouse button pulls.

The upper-arm wave: One of the hardest hit areas of a heavy woman is her upper arms. Because they often lack muscle tone, they tend to flap around like the thing that dangles from under a turkey's neck. You can hear your upper arms telling you to lose weight every time a strong wind blows and they slap you in the face.

The inner-thigh rub: Inner thighs are the loudest part of your anatomy, especially when you wear corduroy pants. In fact, if you strap two sticks on the inside seams, there's enough friction to get them to ignite. This rubbing sound (also known as a "chub rub" for those in the know) is actually your inner thighs screaming at you with every step you take to start a diet. I know that after I've spent a day binging on a tub of frozen Cool Whip, my neighbor calls me to see if I can keep the roar down to a whimper.

The belly overhang: We all know what I'm talking about here, don't we, gals? We zip up our pants and have what seems to be a beached walrus hanging over our waistbands.

Back fat: I never even knew that a back could actually grow fat, but once I was pregnant, I found out about it firsthand. If ever I see myself from behind in a mirror, it looks as if my bra is being swallowed up like bacteria being engulfed by a white blood cell.

Your fingers: I have one unmistakable way of knowing that I've gained weight: my fingers get puffy and I can't seem to take off my ring. I know it doesn't sound like much of a problem, but I have this fear that one day I'll be held up, and the robber will shoot me because I can't get my ring off. I have a bigger fear that one day they'll discover that there's no such thing as PMS, and this is just the way I really am. Either way, my puffy fingers taunt me to slim down.

Your knees and lower back: With every step you take and every stair you climb, these achy parts scream at you for making them work so much harder than they should have to. These pissed-off parts are the unhappy union workers of your body, and they've begun to strike!

It's hard to ignore your "body language," especially when all the various parts are talking to you at once. When I was potty-training my daughter I used to tell her all the time to listen to her body. Of course that didn't stop her from piddling everywhere we went (it seemed not only didn't she listen to her body, she didn't pay a heck of a lot of attention to me either). But if you choose to, you can listen to your various body parts and stock up on carrot sticks. Or you can simply ignore their complaints the same way you do when your parents nag you about wanting grandkids before they're too old to pick them up.

No Smoke, No Wanna Look in Mirrors

Another way to be motivated to start a diet is to stop smoking. Some studies have shown that quitting smoking is more difficult than quitting heroine, cocaine, or that need to squeeze a nasty blackhead that grows on your nose. Some accomplished the feat of quitting by using the patch; others did it by going cold turkey; and still others by staple-gunning their lips together. Chances are these people struggled through strong nicotine fits and even stronger battles with their spouses caused by these nicotine fits. But in the end, they worked through the pain and came out on the other side breathing easier, and smelling much less like a stinky ashtray.

Unfortunately, although these strong individuals did add years to their lives, they may have also added pounds to their figure! Studies show that the amount of weight a person will gain after he or she stops smoking is in direct proportion to how long the person smoked in the first place. The longer the addiction, the longer the belt needs to be in order to go around the waist.

Cigarettes are actually an amazing weight-control device. Nicotine suppresses the appetite and, by raising the heart rate, increases the metabolism. It fills the mouth with smoke and dulls the taste buds so that even a Tastykake fails to live up to its name.

If you've just quit smoking, I wouldn't recommend that you start a diet too soon. I'd suggest that you wait at least six months before you start any other additional withdrawal process. I don't smoke, but the stress of dieting alone makes even me want to light up from time to time.

If you've recently quit smoking, or you're still carrying around extra weight from when you stopped years ago, you're not alone. Everyone turns to food when they break an addictive habit (except for maybe those pod people who have the ability to go to Dairy Queen and simply order a cup of coffee). In fact, here's a list that's put together by the professional team of MMI (me, myself, and I) that breaks down exactly how much weight one can expect to gain while kicking any nasty habit:

1. Cigarette smoking: 10 to 20 pounds
2. Heroin: 30 pounds (including all the brain matter that was lost)
3. Shoe addiction: 5 pounds (but most of it's the extra cash that the former addict will now have in her pocket)
4. Bad Boys: 180 pounds (the approximate weight of the bad boy they were finally able to dump)

I know that carrying around extra weight doesn't make you feel too good about yourself, and may even make you want to start smoking again just so that you'll look better in your Seven jeans. But there is another way to look at it. What you weigh once you quit smoking is probably what you'd weigh if you never started smoking in the first place. And if you think that it may be healthier to be a smoker than to be overweight, let me tell you something. The truth is that you'd have to be about 100 to 150 pounds overweight, depending on your frame, to equal the health risks of being a smoker.

Now that you've stopped smoking in order to lead a healthier life, or in order to get your nagging spouse off your back, you may be motivated to take the next step and lose some of the extra weight that you've gained. Just be realistic about your goal weight. It shouldn't be what you weighed when you were a smoker, because that was an unnatural weight to begin with. You can just throw that dream away, along with your hopes of ever seeing Destiny's Child together in concert or the hope of marrying that great boyfriend to whom you gave the marry-me-or-leave ultimatum.

Growing Up . . . and Out!

I'm just over forty years old, and as I've always heard would happen, my metabolism has started to slow down. Actually, it's been slowing down a little bit every year, but this year, it's slowed down as much as the sales at Wendy's after someone found a finger in their chili. (By the way, it turned out the finger was cut off on purpose, so please don't avoid Wendy's. They make an awesome burger!)

When I was a kid, I could eat whatever I wanted to and would pretty much stay at the same weight. And trust me, I used to eat a lot. By all measures, I should weigh as much as a Dodge Caravan. But now I seem to gain weight no matter what I eat, and if I diet, the weight comes off with the speed of an airport security line on a holiday weekend.

But at least I had skinny years. Now there's an epidemic of overweight children, and I can't imagine how heavy these kids are going to be when they hit my age. When I was a kid there were very few heavy children. In the Stone Age years of my youth, we didn't have computers or video games. To turn on the TV, we actually had to get off our tushies and walk over to the set. We couldn't buy candy and soda at school, and they hadn't even invented the word "supersized."

But now my childhood is over and I too am turning channels without getting up. In fact, I look for any excuse not to get up at all. Because of this, and my slower metabolism, my body is changing. I'm getting fat in places that I never used to before, and it's causing my whole body to sag. My once tight ass is hanging somewhere around my knee area, and I'm forced to buy jeans that they politely call "relaxed fit."

So if you're over forty and you notice these changes as well, it just may be the motivational factor that you'll need to lose weight. There are some different ways to go about weight loss at this age, which you'll learn in Chapter 7. Dieting and exercise have changed a lot over the years, and these changes are for the better. So let's take advantage of these advances now that we're at an age when we pee on ourselves when we cough.

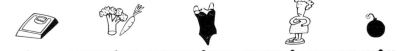

chapter two

why we live to eat
and eat and eat

In theory, it sounds so easy. Simply eat less food and you'll lose weight. But things are rarely as easy as they seem. Telling a heavy person to just stop overeating is like telling an alcoholic to stop drinking, a smoker to stop smoking, or Charlie Sheen to stop using prostitutes. It just doesn't work that way. When you think about it, all the popular diets throughout history have used this same oversimplified theory to get you to shed pounds. They tell you different versions of the same thing: "Limit your intake of processed food." "Don't eat sugar." "Consume less fat." Their theories are all quite valid and seem so easy to follow. But for a variety of reasons, following a diet is one of those things that is much easier said than done.

I know that many a morning, I'll lie in bed and tell myself that today will be the day that I'll change my life. Today I'll be strong and avoid temptation, and once and for all, finally stick to a diet. I mentally plan out the meals for the day and get revved up to start my new leaner life. But

25

when I get to the kitchen and open the fridge, something goes horribly awry. I see the grapefruit and slice of wheat-berry bread that I had planned to eat, but somehow, as if controlled by aliens, or the ghost of Orson Welles, I grab the bag of buttermilk biscuits and the vat of creamy butter, and soon, I'm throwing a party in my mouth. Once I devour the biscuits, I figure I've already blown my diet for the day so I head back to the fridge and attack it like paparazzi descending on a celebrity wedding.

After the invasion, I stand back and assess the damage. In twenty minutes I have eaten enough calories to sustain a grizzly bear through a long, hard winter. I don't understand what has gone wrong. Where did all my determination go? How can I expect myself to lose weight when I couldn't even stick to a diet past one lousy meal? And, as I can tell by your nod of agreement, I'm not the only one who has had this type of experience. Yes, this same scenario is played out in kitchens all around the world every single morning, although the biscuits may be replaced by scones, baguettes, tortillas, or naan.

There are many reasons why following a diet is harder than following what the hell Ozzy Osbourne is saying. No longer do we eat to live; we now live to eat, and many of us live life to its fullest. So if you're having a hard time sticking to your diet, don't blame yourself, especially when there are so many other things to blame. Let's take a look at some of the many reasons why dieting is never as easy as it seems.

Food Is All Around

There's an old saying that would seem to help the average dieter: out of sight, out of mind. But in today's society, escaping food is a physical impossibility. Everywhere we turn we're never far from a tempting tidbit, a decadent dessert, or a naughty no-no. You never realize just how much you're surrounded by food until you go on a diet (or how often food commercials are on TV until you're home with the stomach flu).

The best way to demonstrate my point is to compare today's culture to that of the most recognizable era in human history, namely, the days of *Little House on the Prairie*. Being overweight was a difficult thing for the average prairie dweller to achieve. Back then, there were no refrigerators stocked with leftover moo shoo. The little schoolhouse didn't serve fried fish sticks and Tater Tots in its cafeteria or have vending machines stocked with Abba-Zaba bars. And Ma never cooked meals like Hamburger Helper or Spam tacos because processed food hadn't been invented yet, which is a good thing, because neither had Tums.

But that was yesteryear and today the opposite is true, for staying thin now is as much of a challenge as finding a parking place at the post office on April 15. And who can blame us? Everywhere we turn we're surrounded by something to eat. And I don't mean containers of red peppers and artichoke hummus. I'm talking about fattening food that has more calories than P. Diddy has bling-bling. You can't pay at a gas station without being tempted by a nukable burrito, a greasy hot dog, or some yummy nachos with the kind of melty cheese that you pump from a vat. You can't get your car washed without having to sit next to a display rack of candies and snacks as you wait for your car to be dried. Heck, you can't even earn a living without having to face yet another coworker's birthday cake with icing so thick it can double as Spackle. Yes, in today's culture, we're reminded of food more often than a teenage boy is reminded of sex . . . and that's saying something!

Because of the amazing quantity of nearby places offering something to eat, you're never far away from your nearest craving. There are coffee shops on every corner that serve blended coffee drinks so decadent, they're like sipping cake through a straw. You can't go to the drugstore without having to walk past its in-house ice-cream shop on your way to the bunion-cream aisle. It seems that with every errand you run, you also run the risk of ruining your diet. Just this morning, I took my car in to be serviced and was greeted not only by my trusty mechanic, but by a tasty box of Krispy Kreme doughnuts as well. Now that's what I call full service!

Just think about how much thinner we'd all be if we had to put some effort into satisfying our craving. As you know, we live in a lazy society with drive-through windows and curbside service that makes it all too easy for us to sit on our ass in our heated leather seats for longer periods of time. Heck, we now even keep mini-refrigerators next to our La-Z-Boy recliners so we can grab a beer without expending even one itty-bitty calorie. It'd be one thing if satisfying out latest craving meant walking a mile to the nearest convenience store or taking a bike ride downtown. At least the lazy part of our brain might win out if getting food involved putting forth the smallest bit of effort. But no. The next thing you know, Hostess is going to sell a line of predigested snack cakes so that our bodies don't have to expend all that energy getting the sugar into our bloodstream.

I'd Rather Eat Dog Food than Diet Food

It's hard to imagine how we ever got into this overweight mess to begin with when Mother Nature is truly an excellent cook. She's provided us with some of the most delicious cuisine available on Earth, and it's not only healthy, but low in calories too. What can taste better than a crisp apple in the fall, or a bowl of sweet berries with farm-fresh milk? But once when we sink our teeth into hot apple pie or a strawberry cheesecake, we find the answer. Yes, it seems there's a whole world of other fabulous cooks out there, like Sara Lee, Marie Callender, and Dolly Madison, who are all capable of kickin' Mother Nature's ass on Iron Chef.

We don't seem to be satisfied with Ms. Nature's cooking for a very long time in our life. True, as babies we're content with our strained carrots and mashed peas. Besides breast milk, it was all we knew. But once we took that first bite of birthday cake, there was no turning back. By school age, our lunches had less fruit and more Fruit Roll-Ups. And by adulthood, the only vegetable we crave is a Bloomin' Onion from Outback Steakhouse. Trying to return to eating whole grains, fruits, vegetables, fish, and chicken is like asking a celebrity to give up his fortune and fame and become a civilian like the rest of us. You'll find that within no time, that celebrity will go crazy and clamor for his old seat at Spagos and a bowl of M&M's separated by color.

When it comes to eating, we've veered far off course from the taste of real food. Our taste buds are so accustomed to imitation crabmeat and processed flour that when we go on a diet, we have to retrain them all over again. Starting off our day with whole wheat toast is quite a feat when we're used to having a cheese Danish. A side dish of a baked potato is never as satisfying as potatoes au gratin. And a cup of steamed rhubarb just isn't the same as a slice of rhubarb pie.

That's why when you go on a diet, you tend to seek out the processed foods instead of fresh—foods like low-fat ice cream and low-cal pizza, which have half the fat and none of the flavor of their full-fat, high-calorie counterparts. You'd think that if science can put a man on the moon and make a douche that makes your privates smell April fresh, they could create a diet food that would provide all the artery-clogging transfatty flavor that we've grown to know and love.

The taste of diet food can be even worse when it's the kind that's geared for a specific diet. For example, there's a whole line of "approved" foods for a low-carb diet, including low-carb pasta, low-carb cereal, and low-carb bread, all of which have the taste of baked cardboard. But surprisingly enough, dieters gulp down these tasteless treats. If you ask me, the companies who make these products are far too lax in their approval process.

It's no wonder that one of the most difficult and challenging parts of sticking to a diet is the actual taste of diet food: Pasta that's made without white flour. Jelly that's made without sugar. Potato chips that are made with something called olestra that can cause cramping, diarrhea, and leaky stools. Yes, diet food can be hard on your taste buds, hard on your stomach, and even hard on your underwear.

You Get What You Pay For

In addition to the aforementioned problems associated with eating healthy, it seems that eating healthy is also quite hard on your wallet. Eating a diet rich in fruits, vegetables, lean meats, and fish may be good for your body, but they cost a heck of a lot more money than the prepackaged processed versions. That's because processed foods usually use cheaper, lower-quality ingredients, mix them together with fillers, by-products, and imitation flavors, and sprinkle them with a good dose of preservatives to make them last longer than the plastic they're packaged in.

Most people learned this fact early on in life—specifically, when they first moved out of their parents' house. For the first time ever, these young adults were now forced to buy their own groceries. They finally realized just how expensive food can be, and why their parents got so mad at them for leaving the refrigerator door open. Unfortunately, this time coincided with their new entry-level-position paycheck. Instead of Mom's smothered pork chops and brisket, all they could afford were foods like Ramen noodles, meat in a can, and other low-cost budget items that stretched their dollars like hot cheese on pizza. The good news is that all the heavy food they ate stuck to their ribs. The bad news is that it also stuck to their hips.

"When I moved into my first place I lived on that neon-colored macaroni and cheese. I'd buy it at the drugstore in a three-pack for next to nothing. I'd mix it with scrambled eggs for breakfast and even made mac 'n' cheese sandwiches with mayo on white bread for lunch. Although this food kept me alive, I'm reminded of those early days every time I look at myself in a three-way mirror."

—Stacy

To prove my point about just how cheap fattening food can really be, just walk into any fast-food restaurant. They have a whole menu's worth of high-calorie food that you can buy for just under a buck. But take that same dollar and go into a non-fast-food restaurant, and that buck will just about cover the tax on a healthy roasted vegetable sandwich. What this means is that if you pay for crap, you'll end up with crap. Okay, bad analogy since no matter what kind of food you eat, you'll end up with crap, but you get my gist.

To prove my point even further, and to provide more entertainment value to this book, I've compiled a list of the prices of fresh food items at my local supermarket and the prices of the more processed, and sometimes more humorous version of the same.

HEALTHY FOOD PRICE	JUNKIER VERSION
One large apple = $1.25	One apple turnover = $0.95
One serving of whitefish = $5.15	One serving of fish sticks = $0.95
One russet potato = $0.90	One small bag potato chips = $0.20
One boneless, skinless chicken breast = $2.15	One order of chicken nuggets = $0.89
One pound fresh crabmeat = $35.99	One pound imitation crab = $5.99
One loaf whole grain bread = $4.19	One loaf white bread = $3.29
One cup of milk = $0.50	One cup of Milk Duds = $0.45
One serving of mixed nuts = $1.50	One serving of doughnuts = $0.45
1 pound red peppers = $2.75	1 pound Red Vines = $1.99

Not only does healthy food cost more to buy at the supermarket, but it can also cost more to buy when you buy it from a diet facility. Several popular diets, including Jenny Craig and NutriSystem, require you to purchase their food. When you break down the cost of each meal, you could buy two Quarter Pounder hamburgers for about the price of one single-serving, pre-packaged whole-wheat pasta primavera.

But the truth is that things are rarely as they seem and yes, while junk food is certainly cheaper to buy than health food, there are many other factors that turn this fact into fiction. If you think about it, just the eventual triple bypass can turn these figures around.

Comfort and Joy, Comfort and Joy

Comfort food is a major reason why dieting can be so damn difficult. As most of us know, food provides us with much more than a way to keep ourselves alive. It also provides us with a great deal of contentment. Whenever we bite into a warm chocolate chip cookie, it's like putting a pair of flannel jammies on our tongue. And when we swallow a buttery spoonful of mashed potatoes, it's like filling our tummies with grandma's kisses. Yes, eating comfort food is a great way to deal with life's daily stresses, and is far tastier than biting our nails or chewing on pencils, or doing any of those other silly things skinny people do that enable them to pass on food when they're stressed.

There's no mystery as to why we turn to comfort food in times of need. Thinking back on your childhood, you'll no doubt remember dozens of times when your parents used food to placate your tears. When you skinned your knee, you were soothed by a bowl of ice cream. When you hit your head, you were handed a cookie. And when you cut your first tooth, you were given a frozen waffle to gnaw on (sure, some of you were given a few drops of whiskey, but that's because your parents thought someone in the house should be tipsy with all that screaming going on). In fact, whenever you needed comfort as a child, you inevitably got a treat shoved in your mouth to calm you down.

To add insult to injury, many of our favorite childhood memories go hand in hand with food. The intoxicating aroma of Sunday night dinner cooking on the stove. That mouth-watering bite of a homemade gingerbread cookie during the holidays. The unbelievable smell of blueberry pie pulled fresh from the oven. It's no wonder why, when we crave comfort as an adult, we reach for foods that remind us of our childhood, like gooey grilled-cheese sandwiches, yummy pot pies, and sweet treats like rice pudding, chocolate cake, and double-thick malted shakes. Mmmm, just thinking about it makes me in desperate need of comfort right now!

In the grown-up world, there are many reasons to return to the days of our youth and to comfort food. Single people need comfort food to relieve them of the stress of feeling lonely. Married people need it to relieve them of the stress of having to put up with living with someone day in and day out. Commuters need it to deal with road rage. And parents need it to deal with screaming rug rats who are forever teething and skinning their knees.

I wish I had a different solution for dealing with these problems, but they've been around as long as the common cold and no one has found a solution for that yet either. Sure, you could try to stop using food as a calming device when your tykes take a tumble. Instead of consoling them with something sticky and creamy, shove a piece of jicama in their mouths, or hand them a healthful plate of wilted greens. I doubt that will calm them down much, but I guess a mouthful of any food would drown out the noise some. Maybe you could start serving up putrid meals on Sunday nights, like creamed chipped beef or liver-and-onion surprise. And instead of gingerbread cookies on Christmas, whip up a batch of ginger and soy cookies. That way when kids get older, they'll have no recourse than to do things like bite their nails or chew on pencils when they're stressed, too. It may not calm them down much, but at least they will look better in jeans when they become grandparents, and after all, isn't that the important thing?

Mind over Cookie Batter

The reason that many people overeat is far more complicated than just the need for comfort. They may have deep psychological issues that are temporarily eased by sticking a pork chop in their pie hole. These issues may have stemmed from an incident that took place many years ago, such as parental abuse or the death of a close family member. Or it may be caused by something that the individual is currently dealing with, such as a loveless marriage or a lack of self-worth. These issues can leave people with a void in their lives that can only be filled with a sausage and cheese Hot Pocket. In these cases, food is used as a way of coping, a way of taking control, and a way of licking wounds while licking away at a double-dip cone.

Frankly, I'm a bit jealous of people who can pinpoint their weight gain to one specific incident. At least that way, after they work through their problem, they won't feel the need to overeat. I've thought back over my childhood many times but found no major issue that would account for my large size. Sure, there was the time my mom forgot me at the ice-skating rink, or the time when my sister teased me in front of all the other kids on the bus about a mole I have on an embarrassing part of my anatomy. But I figure those minor things only account for the extra weight I have on my left calf. I'm still struggling to recall something else that would rationalize the size of my hips.

If you think you have a psychological reason for being overweight, you could spend years in analysis going over your childhood and discussing your feelings about your mother, but that's certainly not a tasty solution. The simple fact is that food is capable of providing us with a sense of temporary fulfillment and peace. And while big-ticket stress items may take years to be dealt with, other more common ones take only one meal.

Here's a list of medicinal groceries for some of the most common emotional issues:

You find out you're the only one in your circle not invited to a party: The right side of the menu from your favorite greasy Chinese place.

He doesn't call: Salted pretzels eaten with an equal amount of chocolate chips in the same mouthful.

Hedoesn't call after you sleep with him: A double-cheese pizza with a stuffed crust.

Missingthe one-day clearance sale by one day: An iced blended mocha with whipped cream and caramel sauce.

Spending the holidays alone: A gallon of cookie dough ice cream.

Spending the holidays with your in-laws: A gallon of cookie dough ice cream with a hot fudge chaser.

And We'll Have Fun, Fun, Fun, until Daddy Takes Our T-Bone Away

In addition to providing comfort, food also provides us with a great deal of entertainment value. And it does so in two very distinct ways. The first is that most social functions seem to revolve around food. Think about it. When was the last time you received an invitation to a "Let's sit around the house and read a good book party" or "Let's celebrate our anniversary by painting the trim in our living room?" Never. Instead we go to cocktail parties that serve drinks with little umbrellas, and "pigs" wrapped in flaky blankets. We attend four-course-meal dinner parties and school picnics that feature burgers and macaroni salad. You can't even attend a funeral without going back to someone's house for a party that has more fixings than a food court.

The other reason that food is seen as a source of entertainment is that it supplies us with something to do whenever we get bored. I'm not sure why it is exactly, but it seems that every minute of every day must be filled by doing something stimulating. If you find yourself just sitting around with nothing to do, your first instinct is to head straight toward the kitchen to get something to eat. It doesn't matter if you're hungry. What matters is whether there's any leftover calzone in the fridge.

Yes, living in today's modern world has many benefits, like portable DVD players, pushup bras, and zit concealers, but it also has one major disadvantage: we're so used to massive amounts of stimulation that we find ourselves craving more and more of it in order to be satisfied. We can't drive our cars without listening to the radio, chatting on our cell phone, and applying mocha-latte lip-gloss. We can't work on our computers without instant messaging our friends and buying a Spider-Man sleeping bag for our nephew's sixth birthday.

Back in the old days, we'd be content to watch the same channel all night long because we were too darn lazy to get up off of our plastic-covered sofa and turn the dial. Now we have a universal remote control with picture-in-picture hi-def screen and Sensurround sound. Still, we need the entertainment factor of stuffing our faces full-a Fritos. Not long ago, people would happily go to silent, black-and-white movies. These days we need computer graphics, special effects, and a $12 box of Sno-Caps.

When you think about it, why is it fun to eat anyway? What's so entertaining about chewing a mouthful of food until it's saturated with enough saliva to make it soft enough

" My husband and I can never agree on a movie. He likes the violent stuff and I go for the romance. Whenever it's his turn to decide I make sure that we at least go to my favorite theater, which serves hot dogs from Pink's. I figure if I have to sit through two hours of explosions, he has to sit through two hours of my explosions later that night from eating all those dogs. "

—Laurie

to swallow? What's the joy in munching away on a can of Pringles? Okay, maybe Pringles isn't the best example, because it really is quite fun to get them to fit on my tongue like a crispy potato blanket. Maybe Ho Hos are a better example, although I do love to peel off the outer chocolaty coating without it breaking and then unroll the cake and lick out the creamy center. Okay, okay, forget what I said. I guess eating food is pretty darn entertaining after all.

Occupational Hazard

Let's face it. There are temptations in every profession known to mankind. If you work in a corporate office, you're tempted to pilfer a few office supplies. If you work in a dermatologist's office, you're tempted to swipe a few tubes of wrinkle cream. And if you work at Baskin-Robbins, you're tempted to try each of the 31 flavors with every shift that you take. At least I would. Yes, working in the food business is by far the most tempting profession of them all, and can make sticking to a diet quite a difficult feat indeed.

I myself have worked in several jobs in the food industry over the years and know firsthand how difficult and fattening that kind of work can be. I've been a waitress at a pizza restaurant, a cook at a roasted chicken fast-food joint, and my favorite job of all, a cashier at a cookie store in a mall, where I had a freezer full of raw cookie dough at my disposal. When I worked there I was in hog heaven, and decided that whenever I pass away, I want to be cremated and have my ashes spread all over that nirvana of a Sub-Zero.

You too may have a job that makes keeping your weight down very challenging. Maybe you have a job as a chef or a

> **"**When I started my job as a bank teller three years ago, I weighed almost twenty pounds less than I do now. I'm sure it doesn't help that I just sit around all day, but the big culprit is the fact that the bank is right next door to a doughnut shop.**"**
>
> —Leslie

waitress, with food just an arm's length away. Maybe you're a checkout clerk at a convenience store surrounded by a display rack of candy bars. Or maybe you work in a profession that requires a lot of traveling and are therefore forced to eat food that starts with the prefix, "Mc." Whatever profession you're in, you find yourself locked in a career in which keeping your girlish figure seems as difficult as not peeking at the office payroll when your boss accidentally leaves it in the copy machine.

I have a job now where I'm often tempted by food. True, I'm a writer and spend most of my day in front of a computer, but my computer is located just steps away from my refrigerator. The way it stands now, whenever I need to replenish my creative juices, I do so with a handful of Lorna Doone cookies, some mini blueberry muffins, or some leftover fried chicken. If you take into account that my average book contains 250 pages, that's a whole lotta juices that need to be replenished.

I'm not saying that sticking to a diet is impossible when you're surrounded by food all day at work; it's only that it can be much more of a challenge. But there are some things that you can do to curb your urge to splurge:

1. Always keep healthy snacks close by like fruit, cut-up veggies, or a bag of whole grain cereal to munch on.

Many healthy snacks now come in individual servings, which makes this much easier to do. And no, a bulk size bag of Doritos is not an individual serving, even though it is just a single bag.

2. Brown-bag it. Make sandwiches with whole grain bread filled with lean meat and fresh veggies that will not only fill you up, but also keep you satisfied a whole lot longer than sugary sweets will. Plus, you can use the brown bag to put over your head so you don't see everyone else eating their much tastier lunches.

3. If you must eat at a fast-food joint that doesn't have any healthy options, chose a kids'-size meal. These miniature versions of supersized meals are actually much closer to an appropriate serving size anyway. And besides, they come with a fun little toy!

4. Make a career move and work in the medical waste removal field, a sewage treatment plant, or some other type of work environment that will make you lose your appetite completely.

You're Gonna Have to Face It, You're Addicted to Grub

Even though I put my full trust in the FDA when it comes to keeping my food and medicine safe, I disagree with them on one vital point. Contrary to their studies and reports, I am convinced that certain foods are just as addictive as certain drugs. I know this because (as I stand up and admit this to the world) I am a sugar-holic. Yes, I have a severe physical need for sweets of any kind each and every day. In fact, my body requires a minimum of 400 grams of the stuff (the equivalent of half a tube of cookie dough) just to make it through the day, twice that much if know I have to fold a fitted sheet.

Although I'm not proud of my condition, I know that I am not alone. I realize that there are many others of you out there who are addicted to sweets, salty food, or anything that contains more grease than a can of WD-40. Granted, our body's addiction to certain foods may not manifest itself the same way that an addiction to a harmful illegal substance would do, but the substance is nonetheless just as addictive. I believe our bodies have the same capacity to crave cocaine as they do carbs, and heroin as much as Ho-Hos. In addition, I think that we build up the same kind of tolerance for our substance of choice and find that we need more and more of it every day in order to satisfy our daily fix. I'll even go so far as to say that if we deny ourselves access to this substance, we will go through the same types of physical withdrawal symptoms as we would with any other addictive substance.

As with all addicts, admitting that you have a problem is not only the most difficult part of the healing process, but also the most important. Although it may be unpleasant, see if you can recognize yourself in any of the following scenarios. If you do, there is a good chance that you, too, are addicted to grub.

1. After going marketing, you load up the back seats with the bags of food. You notice the box of Mallomars sitting right on top of one of the bags, but you try to be strong. Unfortunately, your willpower has the strength of a coma victim. As you reach the first light, you contort your body into a position usually reserved for a Cirque du Soleil performer in order to grab the box. You ignore the green light and the honking traffic behind you, and

rip open the box with your teeth. By the time you reach your driveway, you're covered with crumbs and have to add Mallomars to your new shopping list.

2. You first-grader brings home a half-eaten Valentine's Day cupcake that she got at her school party, and asks if she can have the rest after dinner. You agree but as you're cooking dinner, you can't get that cupcake out of your mind. You see her hypnotized in front of *Blue's Clues*, so you pop the remainder of the cupcake in your mouth in one delicious bite. After dinner, you tell your kid that the dog must have eaten your cupcake and that the reason that your teeth are stained red is because you bought some new cheap lipstick.

3. You're at a wedding reception in front of the enormous dessert buffet. You've eaten so many petits fours that you can feel your intestines pushing their way through your newfound umbilical hernia. You swear to yourself that you'll never eat another sweet again, but somehow manage to chow down another plate of treats after they throw the bouquet.

You wonder how you got to this point in the first place. Like most addictions, it no doubt began with peer pressure. I know it did for me. "Go ahead, buy another box of Girl Scout Cookies. It's for a good cause." So I did. But the problem started when I ate the whole box of Thin Mints before I could put them in the freezer, where all Thin Mints legally need to be stored. As time went on, I moved on to harder stuff, like raw cookie dough and Double Stuf Oreo cookies. I'd sit back in my chair with a contented look on my face and schmutz all over my shirt. But I didn't care. I was happy. A little sick to my stomach, but happy.

After time, I bottomed out. I had a mouthful of cavities and my willpower had wrinkled up like an old man's testicles. I denied myself nothing and in return, my desire was out of control. I'd spend my whole day thinking about food and planning my day around which drive-throughs were on my way to work and which desserts I wanted to thaw. Yes, my friend, I became an addict. And like a true addict, I tried to keep my addiction a secret. I'd tell my friends and family at a party that I only wanted a little salad, but omit the part about how I downed a box of yogurt-covered raisins on the drive over.

If you're an addict and you want to get help, what do you do? You can't go cold turkey the way other addicts do, unless your idea of cold turkey is to swap out sweets for lean deli meat. The best thing you can do is try Overeaters Anonymous and learn the twelve steps to healthier eating. Actually, I'm in desperate need of a program like this because right now, I'm about twelve steps away from an opened can of whipped frosting.

The Bigger the Badder

These days, people like things big. We like big-screen TVs, giant boom boxes, and cars that are so enormous, they have more square footage than the average living room. We also like our meals big. Gone are the days of trendy spa food. Today a meal isn't really a meal until it contains enough food to satisfy the Jolly Green Giant. Just look around you. Jumbo-size hot dogs, supersized meals, and soft-drink cups that are five times larger than the average bladder.

One of the best examples of this modern-day magnification is the candy bar. I remember when I was a kid, a candy bar was not much bigger than a concert ticket. Today it's the size of a loaf of French bread. The next time you find yourself walking down the candy aisle (which is the happiest place on earth as far as I'm concerned), take a look at the size of a Butterfinger bar. The only way to ever lose weight with those things is if you buy two and use them as dumbbells.

Of course the problem with today's enormous portion size is that eating a meal makes your stomach blow up like . . . well, like something that blows up to an enormous size. Forgive me, I've written a lot of jokes up till now and I guess I need a moment to regroup. Eating to excess becomes a Catch-22. Your stomach stretches out after each large meal, forcing it to want even more food the next time in order to fill itself up. This cycle can go on and on and on until your stomach stretches out like the elastic in your hubby's boxer shorts (there, I'm back!).

Just the other day I went to a Superbowl party where all the men were watching TV and all the women were around the food table discussing the stupidity of football. That night I ate myself sick on chimichangas. (Isn't that a great name? I'm tempted to get myself a dog just so I can name it Chimichanga. I also like the name Medula Oblongata, but only if it's a girl.) I was so full, yet I somehow managed to find room in my stomach to fit in just one more. It seems that our stomachs are like little clown cars that can accommodate an endless stream of clowns, or in this case, chimichangas.

Whenever you make packaged food like cereal or instant rice, you can see firsthand just how out of control a portion size has truly become. For instance, did you know that a serving size of rice is only half a cup? So is a serving size of ice cream. I don't know about you, but I eat an average serving size with every spoonful. I can eat an enormous quantity of food without even breaking a sweat. In fact, I have that talent listed on my resume under "Special Skills."

The next time you sit down to dinner, you should calculate exactly how many serving sizes you're actually eating. If you're anything like me, you'll find that you're eating enough to feed the Waltons. If you don't know what constitutes an actual serving size, here are some guidelines:

1. A serving size of cooked pasta, rice, or cereal is enough to fit inside the plastic bottle that comes in a box of hair dye.

2. A serving size of a side dish like mashed potatoes or coleslaw is about the size of a palmful of styling mousse.

3. A serving size of meat, chicken, or fish is about the length and width of an iPod . . . but not the ittybitty nano kind, because that'd just be mean.

4. A serving size of cheese is about the size of a tube of lipstick.

5. A serving size of pretzels or chips is enough to fill the cup of a 34B bra.

It's Just Emotion That's Makin' Me Hungry

This is my problem. Whenever I'm emotional, I eat. Whenever my daughter's having a tantrum, I reach for a frosted granola bar. If I'm sad about a sick pet, I reach for a bag of honey mustard pretzels. And if I'm mad at my husband because he's once again put dirty dishes into the clean dishwasher, I reach for one of last night's leftover chicken legs. Not so much because I'm hungry, but because the sturdy bone makes an excellent weapon to pound him over the head with. It seems that no matter what emotion I'm experiencing, food just helps me deal with it so much better. Life is hard, so I eat.

Maybe you can relate. Maybe when you're faced with a problem, you put a handful of Funyuns in your face. This wouldn't be such an issue if women didn't spend so much of their day faced with problems. But life seems to be like an endless sand hill of tedious things to do, and once you conquer them all and get to the top of the pile, you find yourself sliding right back down to the bottom. The minute you finish the last load of laundry, your husband puts his stinky gym clothes in the hamper. As soon as you vacuum the living room, your daughter takes off her shoes and pours out half the sandbox on the rug. Never in my life have I had a clean house, a clean car, a cleaned-out purse, and a blank to-do list all at the same time.

I envy those women who don't use food to help them deal with their stress. You know the ones I'm talking about. The kind who say they're too nervous to eat or too mad to even think about food. I can never understand someone like that. How is one too emotional to eat? That's like being so upset, you forget to inhale. It's like trying to grasp the concept of infinity, or fathom what Britney ever saw in Kevin. I just can't seem to wrap my brain around it.

If you're an emotional eater like I am, you can expect to have a more difficult time following any diet plan. That's because we live in a stressful world filled with deadlines, due dates, and hence, Ding Dongs.

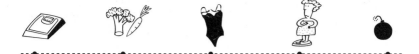

chapter three

the real skinny behind diets

Because of the epidemic number of obese people these days, there is also an epidemic number of diet books. Walk into any bookstore across America today and I bet you'll find a display table covered with newly released titles. There'll no doubt be diet books written by doctors, nutritionists, clinics, and at least one that's written by a Hollywood celebrity with a body so beautiful, it could only have been achieved with a personal trainer, an in-house cook, and monthly liposuction.

Some of these diet books promise quick weight loss. Others swear that if you follow their program, you'll never have to diet again. Still others require that you diet only three hours a day. If you ask me, the only thing that you'll lose if you buy one of these books is $24.95 plus tax.

I'll bet that somewhere on your own bookshelf at home, you have a collection of diet books that you've collected over the years. My guess is that you have some version of a low-carb diet, another one that stresses food combining, and if you're old enough to have owned a pair of Wallabees, one that includes a nauseating amount of grapefruit. Yes, over the years there has been a wide assortment of diet books to choose from, all of which reveal the same mysterious weight-loss secret: if you eat fewer calories than your body burns off, you'll end up losing weight.

Let's face it, if followed correctly, most all diets out there will cause you to drop some pounds, but what these books fail to mention are some of the negative aspects of the diets that are associated with them. These diets somehow omit these "minor" details in the same manner that no one bothers to tell a pregnant woman that she may poop on the delivery room table. In both cases, people feel that some things are better left unsaid. So allow me the honor of filling you in on the real skinny behind some of today's most popular diets.

The Meat of the Matter

The biggest diet sensation of the new millennium has got to be the Atkins Diet, or any similar version of it, which allows you to stuff yourself full of meat and fatty proteins, but greatly restricts the amount of carbohydrates you can consume. Even though the Atkins Diet was introduced back in 1972, it seemed to gain a huge momentum at the turn of this century, along with Uggs, blackhead strips, and feminine napkins with wings. True, it may have lost some steam over the past few years, but it's still quite popular.

The basic premise behind the Atkins Diet is the belief that the body metabolizes carbohydrates first, so if you restrict your intake of carbohydrates, your body will burn fat. Many people saw this diet as the answer to their dreams, because for once in their dieting life, they didn't have to count calories or eat dainty portions of food. Instead, they could stuff themselves full of their favorite forms of protein and fats and still watch the pounds melt away.

Because of the success of this diet, the whole country seemed to go carb crazy. Suddenly, everyone seemed to be watching their intake of carbohydrates. Food manufacturers were making low-carb versions of high-carb products like bread and pasta. Restaurants were serving Atkins-approved meals. Fast-food joints were offering "protein style" versions of burgers and sandwiches, in which the bun was replaced by lettuce leaves. Even candy makers were creating low-carb sweets so as not to be left out of the loop.

I'm the kind of person who follows trends, which is why, at this moment, I'm wearing Uggs, a blackhead strip, and a winged napkin. It's also why I was one of the millions of people who went on this diet. I ate a typical breakfast of a cheese omelet drenched with butter. Lunch was a huge salad with deli meat, avocado, bacon, cheese, and creamy dressing. You'd think I'd be fine, but by the time dinner rolled around, I was craving carbohydrates more than David Cassidy craves the good old days. I looked around the kitchen for something I could eat that would satisfy my desire, but there was nothing to be found. I craved bread, not brisket. Noodles, not nuts. And no amount of sweet sausage would ever satisfy my sweet tooth.

I thought the solution would be to eat a low-carbohydrate version of my favorite foods, so I headed down to my local low-carb market (having these specialty stores nearby is a huge benefit of living in LA and almost makes up for the heart-stopping earthquakes). Unfortunately, when I ate these foods, they all fell short of the original. The crust of the low-carb pizza was chewy. The low-carb chips had a horrible aftertaste. The low-carb pasta was almost unpalatable, and believe me, I have a very strong palate. You could crack a walnut on that thing.

But by far the worst offender was the low-carb desserts. It's not so much that they tasted bad, it's that they had replaced the sugar with an alternative called Splenda. Some people have no problem with Splenda, but others, like me, have a more delicate system. We find that eating Splenda turns our colons into methane factories and creates an enormous amount of toxic gas.

But the problems don't stop there. Besides the intense cravings and the intense gas, there are many other evils to deal with. For one thing, the Atkins diet can also cause a lot of constipation. As you can imagine, when you omit high-fiber foods from your diet, such as whole grains, fruits and certain veggies, your number one problem is going number two. Another problem with the Atkins Diet is that it can cause really stinky breath. I can always tell an Atkins dieter within just a few words. Still another fault is that the diet can be quite costly because you have to buy so much meat. And finally, like so many other diets, this low-carb sensation can also cause severe irritability and bitchiness.

Don't get me wrong; the Atkins Diet can make you lose a tremendous amount of weight. On my first week alone I got rid of 168 pounds, but this was mostly due to the fact that my husband moved into the other room to get away from all my Splenda gas. I am sure that if you stick to the diet, you'll find that the weight will come off rather quickly. The problem, of course, is actually sticking to the diet if you love carbohydrates like bread and sugar. When you finally do give in to the carb craving, it's impossible to stop. You've denied yourself this wonderful pleasure for so long that you just can't seem to get your fill. You're like a newly released Martha Stewart loading up at a tag sale in the Hamptons.

If you do decide to go on the Atkins Diet despite all of the downfalls that I've mentioned, I have a few suggestions that might make the experience easier for you.

1. Try to substitute veggies for carbs whenever you can, just as they do with the "protein-style" burgers. For instance, try cutting a red pepper in half and filling it full of taco fixings. It makes for a crunchy, Atkins-approved shell. You can also use endive leaves to replace potato chips for dips. Go down the produce aisle and be creative.

2. Keep a steady supply of Atkins-approved snacks with you at all times. I used to carry around a bag of nuts and jerky in my purse in case I got hungry on the road. Even though the world is carb crazy, it's still hard to find a place to pull over and grab a quick rib eye.

3. If you miss having sweets, get a few bags of frozen berries (blueberry is my favorite) to keep in your freezer. In fact, if you put some in a bowl and sprinkle them with a touch of cocoa powder and really use your imagination, they taste a bit like chocolate-covered raisins.

4. If you're about to eat Splenda for the first time, I suggest that you first move all of your houseplants outside, just in case you too, have a delicate system!

You're in the Zone

I, like many of you, have a copy of *The Zone Diet* on my bookshelf. It's no wonder; it's probably one of the most popular diet books in recent years. I bought my copy years ago because—well, this is a bit embarrassing to admit—because I read that Jennifer Aniston followed the Zone Diet. I truly believed that underneath my many layers of fat, I have the same body type that she does. I have vague memory flashes of what my body used to look like before I ruined it in college with the self-serve ice-cream station at the commons. I figured that if Jennifer could uncover her thinner self with the Zone, then so could I.

In a nutshell, the Zone Diet, created by Dr. Barry Sears, advocates eating meals that are in a certain proportion. He suggests that each plate of food should contain 40 percent of its calories from carbohydrates, 30 percent from protein, and the remaining 30 percent from fat. That ratio is not just reserved for your basic three meals a day. Even snacks have to follow this same 40-30-30 formula. Dr. Sears believes that when you eat in this manner, you allow your body to perform at its peak, hence, be in the "Zone." This supposedly gives you maximum energy and maximum weight loss, but as I found out, it can give you maximum headaches as well.

When I first started my diet, I was quite gung ho about it. It sounded so good on paper, and in fact, almost too good to be true. I went to the market and loaded up on Zone-approved food like hummus and eggs. But it didn't take long before I found out that putting together a plate of food that attained this 40-30-30 ratio involved an advanced degree in mathematics. Then it hit me why the diet works so well. You have to exert so much effort putting together a meal that's in the Zone that it's not really worth it.

Another problem that I had with the Zone was that I found the portion size to be incredibly small. In fact, I have a friend who recently went on the diet, and chose to use a service that delivered premade, Zone-appropriate food directly to her door. On the first day, she ate her breakfast and figured that she must not have received the rest of the food for the day. When she called the company, she discovered that she actually had eaten the food for the whole day in one meal!

When you're on the Zone Diet, you not only have to say goodbye to big portions and desserts, but you also have to say goodbye to some unexpected items as well, such as caffeine and artificial sweeteners. You can also forget about grabbing a quick snack anymore (unless it's one of those pre-measured Zone bars) because you have to spend more time measuring out your 40-30-30 ratio than you'll spend eating it. And you also can say goodbye to eating out at most restaurants, because you don't have much control over the portion size, how much oil is used, and the exact 40-30-30 ratio.

Although sticking with the diet should allow you to lose a few dress sizes, there is one claim to the diet that I find very hard to believe. Dr. Sears states that one of the benefits of the Zone Diet is that it can actually slow down the aging process. I don't know if that's actually true or if life just *seems* a whole lot longer when you spend most of your day lamenting over the carbohydrate, protein, and fat ratio of every morsel of food that you put in your mouth.

Shake It Up

At first, the idea of going on Slim-Fast sounds inspirational. Who doesn't love the notion of losing weight by sucking down chocolate shakes all day? But as the old adage says, if it sounds too good to be true, it usually is (unless of course you're talking about the taste of peanut butter and chocolate together, because that's just plain heaven!). The reason that this particular example is too good to be true is that Slim-Fast shakes taste nothing like those thick and creamy frozen concoctions we all know and love. In fact, calling a Slim-Fast drink a milk shake is like calling one of those hairless cats a cat. It simply isn't right.

But if you're looking for a diet that's simple, easy to follow, and doesn't make you count calories or carbohydrates, then the Slim-Fast plan is the diet for you. The way it works is easy. You simply replace two of your meals with a Slim-Fast shake, eat three healthy snacks like fruit or nuts, and have one sensible meal. This should keep your daily caloric intake to about 1,200–1,500 calories. They advise that your one meal consist of healthy, portioned-controlled food and that you exercise for thirty minutes a day. Sounds simple, huh? Not really.

The first problem you'll encounter is that you actually have to drink the stuff. Once you pop open the lid, you'll see what I mean, for even the smell of the drink is pretty nasty in my opinion. But it's nothing compared to the taste. The chocolate shake tastes like chocolate in the same way that steel wool feels like wool. If anything, I think the drink tastes more like metal than something sweet. It's as if they mixed the shake with a handful of old pennies and let them ferment for a very long time.

I do warn you that if you are going to try the diet, you should definitely keep the shakes in the refrigerator. The colder they are, the better they'll taste. In fact, maybe you should stick them in the deep freeze and just lick them throughout the day. I also warn you that Slim-Fast shakes contain a lot of fiber, so they can cause a lot of gas. In addition, they're sweetened with Splenda, so when you combine that with the gas you'll get from the fiber, you'll probably be able to propel yourself into space with one single toot.

As you can imagine, drinking an 11-ounce drink isn't nearly as filling as eating a real meal. It wouldn't be so bad if you could mix the shake together with, let's say, a Key lime pie. Lacking that, I tend to get hungry quite quickly after drinking them. If you enjoy a lot of variety, Slim-Fast does deliver. In fact, the plan has an overwhelming array of choices, from different flavors to smoothies and snacks. This may be a problem for people who, like me, struggle over simple decisions like paper or plastic.

But if you can get past the gas, the hunger, the choices, and the taste, the diet really does work. And who knows, maybe you won't find the taste of the thing so bad. When you think about it, there are those who have been stranded for days who were even forced to drink their own urine. I guess when you're hungry enough, you'll eat just about anything.

Cyberdiet

We live in an era when you can log on to your computer and order anything from a book to a boyfriend, an air conditioner to an automobile, and a sex toy to a sex change. And if it's a smaller waistline you're after, you can point and click your way to that as well. That's because cyberspace offers many different Web sites that allow you to simply dial up and diet.

The big kahuna of all the online dieting Web sites is called eDiets.com. The eDiets site offers its own special diet plan, which is based on a calorie-controlled system. Or, if you prefer, you can use the services of eDiets to help you succeed with most every other major diet plan available, from Atkins to the Zone.

Yes, eDiets is plump full of ways to get rid of your extra plump. For one thing, the plans are personalized. When you log on, you're asked to answer some basic questions about your height, age, and weight so that the eDiets folks can give you an individualized diet plan along with meal suggestions, recipes, and even shopping lists. They can also offer substitute foods if you have a certain food allergy or think lima beans are just plain icky. They can even personalize your diet to your specific eating habits and weight-loss goals. Although all of these benefits are great, I think that the best part about eDiets is that you don't have to weigh yourself in front of another human being, or sit through a thirty-minute meeting in which you discuss the evils of butter.

But, like anything else in life, there is a price to pay. First of all, be wary when you sign up for extras like the vast selection of different newsletters and diet horoscopes, because they'll fill up your e-mail folder faster than ads for Viagra do. And unlike other cybersites, such as Amazon and eBay, eDiets requires that you pay a weekly membership fee. For an additional charge, you can get extras like Oprah's cybertrainer, and twenty-four-hour support. Personally, I don't really see how someone can find much support in cyberspace. I need the help of an actual person to talk me down from that slice of three-layer cake.

But if you're the kind of person who doesn't like to travel to meetings, doesn't like to choose your meals for yourself, and doesn't like to be in the company of other human beings, eDiets is a perfect solution for you. That is, if you're computer savvy. Me, I get frazzled by all the pop-up ads and the constant computer freezes, and when the printer says there isn't enough paper when I know full well that I put a stack in just moments ago. The stress caused by technology makes me make a beeline for the brownies and call it a day.

Sugar Busters!

When I first heard about the Sugar Busters! Diet, I was disgusted by the whole idea behind it. For me, a life without sugar is no life at all. In fact, I consider sugar to be one of my oldest and dearest friends. Sugar and I met back at my first birthday party, when I had a fistful of princess cake, and we've been best pals ever since. Sugar's been there for me when I've been bored or nervous, and has provided me with a great deal of comfort during bad hair days and bad breakups. To be honest, I'd have an easier time giving up sex than Suzy-Q's.

Even with my strong feelings on the matter, I do see the logic behind Sugar Busters! and diets like it. I'm no dummy, and I realize that, as much as I love my sugary sensations, they're one of the most concentrated forms of calories and carbohydrates, and are personally responsible for my primeval fear of cinch belts. Adding insult to injury, the Sugar Busters! Diet restricts other foods besides just table sugar. Yes, this diet also forbids certain fruits and vegetables, such as corn, beets, and carrots, that have a higher glycemic index—basically, a measure of how much sugar a certain food has—than do most other kinds of produce. Sugar Busters! also restricts some of the most delicious and comforting starches, including white potatoes, white rice, white breads, and white pastas. As you can imagine, the first week or so of the diet can be excruciating to follow if you're a sugar and bread fan. It's like an addict giving up a fix or Joan Rivers giving up plastic surgery.

Not to say that I'm focusing on the positive (God forbid that I ever do that), but I did find *The Sugar Busters! Diet Book* to be one of the easiest diet books to understand. The font is large in size and the words are easy to understand without attaining a medical degree or watching a dozen episodes of *ER*. In fact, the only way this book could be even more entertaining would be if they threw in a few illustrations of dancing vegetables. In addition, the Sugar Buster! diet is relatively easy to follow and best of all, you're allowed to have wine on the diet as long as you drink it on a full stomach (they believe that the sugar in the wine is absorbed slower in this manner). The book also contains some tasty recipes and many interesting food trivia facts. Although you may find some of these facts to be fascinating, don't be surprised if you drive away your friends and family with your newfound knowledge. Sure, after following the diet, you'll be able to shop at stores like The Limited instead of Lane Bryant, but people will be so sick of your trivia, you won't get invited to parties anymore anyway.

"Lettuce" Lose Weight

Although the Cabbage Soup Diet has been around for quite a while, it's still worth mentioning because, even today, people use it for a quick weight-loss plan. When I was at my very first job, many years ago, a coworker raved about the miracle of this diet. She went on and on about how she lost 10 pounds in seven days. The diet

> **"**When I went on the Cabbage Soup Diet I lived for the day when I was allowed to have one baked potato. I went to three different stores until I found one that must have weighed like four pounds and could double as a doorstop.**"**
>
> —Mary

sounded perfect for me. Not only did I need to lose a good 10 pounds myself, but it was dirt cheap to follow. I was barely making enough money at the time to afford the basics in life, such as food, rent, and Chanel lipstick (a girl has needs). Although everyone was a bit nervous about going on such a strict diet, the whole office agreed to go on the diet together, so the coworker made copies of it and passed it around. We all sat at our desks anxiously awaiting our copy as if it were the results of a pregnancy test.

As it turns out, the Cabbage Soup Diet is a very simple diet to follow. All I did was make a big—and I mean *big*— pot of soup, which contained low-calorie vegetables like cabbage, onions, green pepper, carrots, tomatoes, and celery. This enormous pot of soup lasted for several days, as did the stench it left in my apartment. This soup was the staple of my everyday existence for seven whole days, but each day I was allowed to include one other type of food such as fruit, meat, bananas, and skim milk. My favorite day of the diet was the one that allowed me to eat brown rice. I looked forward to that day as if it were a European vacation.

It wasn't long into the first day that I realized how grateful I was that my whole office was going on this diet together. Not only was it nice to have so much support, but more important, it was wonderful that there were so many other people to blame when I had to fart. Unlike diets that limit your fiber intake, the Cabbage Soup Diet is like eating a big bowl of sawdust. Therefore, you can expect gas levels to rival those of the pumps at your local Exxon station.

Another reason that I was so glad our whole office went through the cabbage experience together is that our boss was never quite sure which one of us was responsible for all of the mistakes that occurred. Since all of us were constantly hungry, we all had the same trouble being able to concentrate, and none of us had enough energy to complete even the simplest of tasks. Be aware that going on the Cabbage Soup Diet may greatly reduce your chance of being voted Employee of the Month.

But after all was said and done, I did end up losing weight on the diet. In fact, those of us who stuck out the diet for the whole seven days lost quite a bit of weight. The problem was that it came back faster than a yeast infection does after a dip in a communal hot tub.

If you're not lucky enough to have a lot of company with you on the diet, here are some suggestions to try to cover up your gas at work:

1. Excuse yourself often to go to the bathroom. Sure, your coworkers will think you've picked up an illegal snorting habit, but it's better than if they found out the truth.

2. If you're lucky enough to have a private office, lock your door, especially if it's your birthday. If your coworkers were to surprise you by walking in your office with a lighted birthday cake, the whole place could explode.

3. Hang out in the lunchroom during mealtime. The place usually reeks of leftover tandoori chicken and various reheated week-old plastic containers.

4. Ask your boss if you could work from home. He'd probably be grateful for the offer.

Health warning: If you do go on this diet, follow their instructions and don't go on it for longer than seven days. I can't imagine that anyone would even think of doing this anyway, but then again, there are those who test to see if a razor is sharp by running their finger along the blade. I guess there's just no accounting for some people.

Blood Is Thicker than Water Weight

If there were ever a diet that seems as silly as the ice-cream-and-peanut-butter diet of the past, it's the Blood Type Diet. This diet is based on the belief that your specific blood type is crucial in determining what kinds of foods you should and shouldn't eat in order to lose weight. This diet is the brain-child of Dr. Peter D'Adamo, a naturopathic physician, who believes that there are "evolutionarily appropriate" diets for people with different blood types. His book, *Eat Right 4 (for) Your Type*, states that someone with an "O" blood type (as found in the oldest evolutionary animals) should not consume wheat or carbohydrate foods, but rather eat a diet that's very high in protein and fat. Those with the "A" type (the next blood type to evolve) should eat a diet rich in carbohydrates. Finally, those with the "B" and "AB" types, which supposedly have developed more recently, have a more "adaptive" intestinal capability and can eat a varied diet, and one that includes dairy foods.

Besides the fact that the logic behind this diet is as hard to believe as Michael Jackson's claim of only having had one nose job, it also has one inherent flaw: Who the hell knows what their blood type is? It's not like human beings are built like Cabbage Patch Kids dolls and come with information tattooed right onto their asses. In order to find out this crucial piece of trivia, we need to get a blood test, another thing that I steer away from at all costs. I'm not going to put myself through the ordeal of going to the doctor's office, waiting an eternity to be seen, getting stabbed with a needle, and then having to fill out a mountainous pile of insurance forms just so I can see whether I should have macaroni or meatloaf for dinner. No way. No how.

Another inherent flaw in the *Eat Right 4 (for) Your Type* diet is that I have yet to find any evidence, other than what's presented in the book, that backs up the theory that blood type determines what a person can eat to lose weight. And if I'm going to go through all the hell of a diet, I'm going to make damn sure that there's a little scientific proof that it actually works.

But if you're not like me and don't care about silly things like blood tests or scientific proof, then by all means, go right ahead and go on the diet. I consider myself to be a person of logic. Things *have* to make sense to me, which is why I can never get past why *Desperate Housewives* cast size-two actresses when the average housewife is actually a size twelve. Maybe that's why today's housewives are so desperate in the first place.

A Walk on the Beach

Dr. Arthur Agatston, a cardiologist, created the South Beach Diet in the mid-1990s. The South Beach Diet soon became one of the most popular diet books of all time and flew off the shelves faster than the tell-all by Scott Peterson's mistress. Personally I think that one of the key reasons for the diet's success is its name. The South Beach diet sounds so exotic and sophisticated, as if it could transform you into someone tan and sexy with long legs in kitty-cat heels. I doubt the book would have been nearly the same success had it been named the South Central LA Diet.

The difference between the South Beach Diet and all the other high-protein diets is that with South Beach, you're allowed to eat carbohydrates, as long as you eat the right kinds. Also, the South Beach diet is broken down into three distinct phases instead of just one plan for the duration. The first phase is quite similar to the Atkins Diet and must be adhered to for two weeks. But instead of being able to gorge yourself on slabs o' bacon and mass quantities of pork fat, the first phase of South Beach stresses eating reasonably sized portions of lean protein like fish and chicken, certain veggies, nonfat or low-fat cheese, nuts, eggs, tofu, and healthy oils (but at least you can wash it all down with coffee or a diet soda). After those first two weeks of torture, you can then add limited amounts of fruits, whole grains, fat-free milk, and yogurt until you reach your goal weight. The third and final phase of the diet is that of maintenance, when you're allowed to eat the greatest variety of food.

Because I'm one of those consumers who believes that if a product is popular, it must be good (which is why I repeatedly use cellulite cream even though my thighs remain as lumpy as ever), I decided to check out the South Beach Diet for myself. I bought the book, shopped for the right foods, and dove right in. I found that much like the stupid cream, the diet wasn't all it was cracked up to be, in this case because there was one flaw that I simply couldn't get past: you had to go through the most difficult phase of the diet first. To me that's like running before you've learned how to walk, singing before you've learned how to speak, or getting rid of that annoying blinking "12:00" before you read the manual for your new DVD player.

Although the South Beach Diet is far less restrictive than Atkins in terms of carbohydrate intake, you have to survive the first two grueling weeks in order to reap the rewards, and how many of us can really stick to a diet for longer than a two-week stretch? Not many. Not many at all. Besides, if I'm going to force myself to stick to a diet for two weeks, I'd rather choose one that lets me eat a platter of rump roast than one skinless chicken breast.

To add insult to diet injury, during the first phase of this diet, you're not allowed to consume alcohol. If they expect you to follow such a torturous program, the least they can do is let you go through it bombed. What *is* South Beach if not a place to relax and pound back a few Pomegranate Mojitos?

> **❝Before I went on this stupid diet, I used to live for the weekend, when I could finally see my boyfriend. Now I live for my nightly two-pack, ninety-calorie, sugar-free Fudgsicle, and my boyfriend comes in at a very distant second.❞**
>
> —Hana

During this first difficult two-week period, you may find that you bite down on your teeth a lot. That's because they're in desperate need of exercise now that your diet is void of crunchy, high-carb foods like cookies and cereal. You also get quite sick and tired of foods like chicken and Canadian bacon. And make sure you budget enough money to buy lots of nonstick cooking spray. Since the diet forbids you to fry your food or sauté anything in butter, there'll be a new girl in your life, and her name is PAM.

Sleeping can also become a big problem when you're on the South Beach Diet. Actually, it can be a difficult problem with any diet, but because South Beach makes you hit the ground running (starving is more like it), your body doesn't have the same amount of time to adjust to the shock caused by eliminating glazed desserts from your diet. If you can, it's best to go on this diet with your bed partner so at least you have someone who's awake with you in the middle of the night to complain to about just how hungry you really are.

Once you make it past the first two weeks of withdrawal, crankiness, and constant fatigue, you're allowed to incorporate a few treats back into your diet. They are limited, though. For example, you're allowed fifteen pistachio nuts, or six mini squares of shredded wheat with six blueberries. You can also incorporate a few desserts into your meals, most of which revolve around mixing ricotta cheese with Splenda, and tossing in five miniature chocolate chips (I did find that if you cheat a bit and bump it up to seven chips, you can have one chip per bite). It's actually a good thing that you can't have more than ten pieces of most snack foods because, after those two difficult weeks of starvation and minimal sleep, you're down to only a few remaining brain cells, which can only handle so much excitement.

The Naked Truth about the Raw Food Diet

Unlike most all other diets, the raw food diet didn't become popular due to a bestselling book. It isn't a business like Jenny Craig or Weight Watchers. Nonetheless, according to Newyorkmetro.com, it's still considered one of the most popular diets today. One of the reasons for this anomaly is that the raw food diet is associated with some hot Hollywood celebrities, including Demi Moore and Woody Harrelson. As you know, anything that's hot in Hollywood influences what we mere mortals do (carry tiny dogs around in a purse), wear (colorful rubber bracelets), and eat (hence this section about raw food).

The raw food diet is really quite simple. You're not allowed to eat anything that's been cooked over 118 degrees. At first I thought that this was the ideal diet, since I know full well that Twinkies require no baking whatsoever. Unfortunately, there's another rule that you must limit your food intake to fruits, vegetables, lean meats, nuts, and juice. That rule really sucked all the fun out of the diet for me, but if you're someone who enjoys a big plate of lawn, then go ahead and check this one out!

In addition to the diet's inherent problem of excluding Twinkies, there's also the fact that it can be an extremely expensive diet to follow. It's one thing to have to buy fresh produce for a diet, but when you add in the cost of foods like carpaccio and sushi-grade tuna, you'll have to get a second job in order to afford Sunday brunch. And if you're not living in a trendy city like Los Angeles or New York, finding a restaurant that serves raw food is as hard as finding a cute guy who will call you when he says he will.

❝ When I went on the raw food diet, I would survive on nothing but vegetable juice and sashimi. It was fine when I was home in Beverly Hills, but when I went to visit my family in Lake Shasta, the only raw fish I could find was at the bait and tackle shop. **❞**

—Hope

To me, the raw food diet seems like a lot of hype. I find that there's no great mystery as to why it causes you to lose a tremendous amount of weight. How could you not lose weight when all you can afford to eat all day is one small bowl of seafood ceviche and a scoop of blueberry mash? Followers of the raw food diet claim that it has other powers besides just curing them of their obesity problem; I've read that it also has been used to cure things like acne, asthma, cancer, and multiple sclerosis. Forgive me for being cynical, but I think that far more people would get sick from this diet than would ever be cured, due to the fact that the food isn't cooked at a high enough temperature to kill off any bacteria and parasites. I know that I'd sure end up dropping a few pounds after I ingested a plateful of E. coli-ridden steak tartare.

Your Friend, Jen

If I had written this book a few years ago, I wouldn't have even included a section about Jenny Craig. Her franchised weight-loss clinics seemed to be about as outdated as Gee Your Hair Smells Terrific shampoo. The Jenny Craig system started a long time ago, 1983 to be precise, but her diet seemed to lack the pizzazz that other, more hip, weight-loss programs had. Jenny Craig didn't have a member of royalty as a spokesperson, and didn't have any catchy jingles.

But Jenny Craig has had a little work done recently and she's looking better than ever! I think that the reason behind this rejuvenation is Kirstie Alley acting as a spokesperson. Kirstie is energetic, fun loving, and has incredible hair no matter how much she weighs. Kirstie has been the CPR of this once dying institution. That's why Jenny Craig is back in the public eye and is as much an icon in today's society as Paris Hilton's chihuahua. But that doesn't mean that her plan has no flaws.

They say that there is no such thing as a free lunch, and Jenny Craig has taken this phrase literally. In fact, her lunches can be very expensive. So can her breakfasts and dinners, for that matter. In fact, many people steer clear of her program because of her hefty membership fee and the price of her food. But if the price of her program is keeping you at bay, I'll let you in on a good money-saving tip that a friend let me in on. Simply take some of her prepackaged food with you to the market and compare her labels against those of some popular brands. You may be surprised to find that Chex cereal is very comparable to Jenny's cereal and that Campbell's soup offers an almost identical version of hers as well.

Jenny is also big on providing support. Unlike Weight Watchers, where there are many people in a room with only one leader, Jenny's support system relies on a one-on-one relationship with your sponsor. Although *her* way provides you with a much more personal support system, it also makes it quite difficult for you to sneak out early or miss more than a session or two.

> **"**I always get intimidated whenever I have to meet with my counselor. She's like some reincarnated Nazi soldier who tells me what I can and cannot do. I can't go out to dinner and I can only eat their food. I've lost almost 75 pounds through their plan, but it may be because of all the stress I go through to be on it.**"**
>
> ——Lisa

I'll admit, I never went on Jenny Craig myself, but I have eaten the food many times over the years. My aunt used to have a closet full of the stuff and I would have it whenever I went to visit as a kid. I used to love going to her house and eating that freeze-dried, packaged food. It wasn't so much that I liked the taste of it; it's just that it made it easy to pretend I was an astronaut.

When it comes to the taste of Jenny's cooking, it's all a crapshoot. I've recently tried her meals and found some to be better than others. But the one thing they all have in common is a small serving size. I found that eating her food was very much like eating Chinese food—you're hungry an hour after you finish your meal.

Besides the expense and taste, I find that the biggest problem with the Jenny Craig diet is that it doesn't train you to prepare your own meals or teach you how to eat out on your own without gaining weight. In fact, the only thing that her meals teach you is how to eat her meals for the rest of your life, which may be the genius behind Jenny Craig's thinking. This Jenny woman is one smart, fat-free cookie!

Somersizing

Suzanne Somers was best known in the 1970s for her bouncing boobs and her bad contract negotiations. In the '80s it was her ThighMaster, and I guess her bouncing boobs. Today, she still has great boobs, but she's most closely associated with her popular diet plan, which she calls Somersizing. The Somersizing plan of weight loss is basically high-protein, high-fat, and low-carbohydrate. Like most all diet promoters today, Somers too advocates eating no sugar or processed food. But her twist on the diet world is that she emphasizes eating foods in a specific combination. Even though there's no scientific proof to back up her theory, she believes that when certain foods are eaten together, their enzymes cancel each other out, thereby stopping digestion and leading to weight loss.

Personally, I have no problem with Suzanne's theory since I'm a big fan of combining foods as well. I always combine a big dollop of butter with my baked potato, some sausage and mushrooms on my pizza, and my favorite combination of all, a box of Milk Duds poured directly into my warm box of movie popcorn. Don't knock it till you try it. It even made Madonna's *Swept Away* worth sitting through!

66 When people ask me how I lost so much weight I have a hard time admitting that I went on Suzanne Somers's diet. It's not the most macho-sounding diet in the world. The Sylvester Stallone diet would be one that was much cooler to admit to. 99

—Stan

After further investigation, I learned that Suzanne Somers's food combinations aren't nearly as much fun as mine are. She firmly believes that you should eat proteins and fats with veggies, carbohydrates with veggies and no fat, proteins and fats separate from carbs, and that you should eat fruit only on an empty stomach. This of course would limit a majority of foods, including traditional sandwiches and pasta dishes (unless they're made with only veggies), and your basic meat-and-potato meals.

Suzanne Somers also has a list of "funky" foods that you should stay away from, including beets, carrots, and bananas, all of which she believes are like little produce candy bars because they contain a lot of sugar. I too have a list of "funky" foods that I stay away from in my fridge, such as green olives that used to be black, and old cheese that's covered with more hair than Robin Williams's back. As you can tell, I'm not big on cleaning out my refrigerator. I rank it lower than all other household chores, including cleaning out my shower drain and taking the gizzards out of a raw chicken.

Although Somersizing is not nearly as well known as diets like Atkins or the Zone, her followers seem to be far more devoted to it than to any other diet plan I've ever seen. In fact, they view Suzanne Somers as the L. Ron Hubbard of the weight-loss world. Her followers look up to her and see her as a survivor who won't go away no matter how much time goes by—like Cher or cockroaches. Those I spoke with even admit that they feel hungry a lot on her diet, but they don't seem to care. They wouldn't dream of cheating on her with any other diet plan. If you ask me, these people are in desperate need of an intervention.

A Pill to Cure Your Ill

How glorious does this sound? Simply pop a pill every day and all of your weight-loss problems will be solved. Within minutes, you won't be hungry and you'll have the energy of a school-age boy with ADHD. Unfortunately, things are never as easy as they sound. Remember Phen-Fen? I sure do. My neighbor lost a great deal of weight on the stuff so I reluctantly decided to start popping those little devils as well. I say "reluctantly" because I don't like taking drugs of any kind. I even used to be against taking aspirin for a headache but changed my mind after seeing how long a headache could linger without those beautiful little gel caps. I know you may think me silly, but what you don't know is that my parents were hippies when I was growing up. They were in group therapy, had themselves Rolfed, and even partook in smoking homegrown pot. So when I went through my turbulent teenage years, my way of rebelling was to become a total nerd. No drugs, alcohol, or lava lamps of any kind.

But once I started taking Phen-Fen, a whole new skinny world opened up to me. For the first time in my adult life, I ate like a thin person. All I wanted for breakfast was a piece of toast. For lunch, it was half a sandwich and a few bites of apple. Dinner consisted of a bowl of Cheerios and half a cookie. This went on for days and I never felt hungry. In no time at all, I lost so much weight that I could have been mistaken for a contestant on *Survivor*.

Then, of course, came all the negative media attention when those who took Phen-Fen seemed to be dying right and left due to heart problems. I hated the thought of giving up my newfound pill-shaped friends and tried to rationalize staying on them. What's a little hole in my heart compared to thin upper arms and a stomach you could bounce a quarter off of? But in the end, I came to my senses and threw the pills in the trash. Within days, my hunger level returned to what it used to be, and the layers of fat grew back like a stubborn ganglion cyst.

How quickly society forgets these kinds of things, which is why we started buying tabloid magazines so soon after Princess Di's tragic death, and why we once again are popping diet pills. This time, however, there's a whole new slew of diet pills that you can buy over the counter. One popular brand is called TrimSpa. The reason that this diet pill is all the rage is because of the enormous weight loss of spokeswoman Anna Nicole Smith. Personally, I think she seemed to have lost a bit of brain matter along with body fat, but nonetheless, the pills are flying off the shelves. There are many other popular brands of diet pills as well, all of which promise to be safe, nonaddicting, and free of ingredients that cause holes in internal organs.

One reason for the success of diet pills is that the ads are so compelling. They often show a "before" picture of a very overweight individual who has been transformed into an "after" who's now thin and sexy. What was once a bloated figure is now beautiful. What was once a saddened face is now sultry. And what used to be a horrible haircut is now a thick mane reminiscent of a Harlequin romance novel cover. How could you not want to suck down these devils like magical M&M's?

But the truth is that not all diet pills are created equal. Some have ingredients that can make your heart race. Others can make you feel nervous or edgy. And don't be misled by a label that says the pills are "all natural." Arsenic is "all natural" too, but I wouldn't want any of it in my diet pill. So if you're in the market for a pill to cure your ill, remember to shop wisely, read labels, and most of all, be realistic. There's no guarantee that any diet pill will give you a thin body or a sexy look. And as for that thick mane of hair? Well, you'll have to look for a pill that lists Rogaine as one of the main ingredients.

NutriSystem

Like Jenny Craig, NutriSystem has been around for a long time, and its image still seems to be stuck in the Dark Ages. The NutriSystem plan is similar to Jenny Craig's in that you have to buy its food—but that's where the similarities end. With Nutriystem, you're not required to meet with any counselors. You're not required to pay any membership fee. And no one checks up on you to see if you're following the diet or doing any exercise. In fact, NutriSystem is an excellent plan for those who are too busy to cook, too lazy to exercise, and too independent to ask for help.

NutriSystem can be quite pricey, costing hundreds of dollars a month for food. I'd understand this expense if you were getting meals prepared by Wolfgang Puck, but in my opinion, the food isn't even that great, especially the desserts. My advice? Steer clear of any of the lemon-flavored diet desserts, because they all taste like furniture polish. When you order your NutriSystem food and it finally arrives, it looks like the kind you'd eat in the army while out in the field. There are powdered eggs and canned meat and boxed meals that resemble frozen food, but require no refrigeration. I don't quite understand how the stuff stays fresh when it's at room temperature. Maybe their weight loss secret is that each meal contains a small dose of salmonella poisoning which tends to kill one's appetite.

One thing that may come as a surprise on the NutriSystem plan is that you have to supplement your prepackaged meals with food you buy at the grocery store, such as fruit, vegetables, and milk. Many consumers have complained about this detail. They feel that since they're paying so much for the food, NutriSystem should throw in a few diced carrots and apple wedges.

My neighbors Carol and Mitch have been on NutriSystem for about three months now. They go online and order the whole month's worth of food at a time and have it delivered directly to their home. When it arrives, it's quite a hefty amount, which they keep stacked high in their garage. When I saw the enormous stacks of food, I knew right away where I was headed when a big earthquake hits. Sure, the canned meat and powdered eggs may not be all that tasty, but it's a whole lot better than eating my dog.

Like all other food delivery systems, NutriSystem's main flaw is that it fails to teach people how to eat once they reach their goal weight. At least that's a flaw from the consumer's point of view. To the people at NutriSystem, it guarantees a lifetime of orders, which may explain why NutriSystem, like Jenny Craig, has been around for as long as it has.

The Grandam of Diets

Weight Watchers has been around longer than any other popular diet plan today. It was started back in the early 1960s by Jean Nidetch, a woman from Queens, who asked some friends and neighbors if they wanted to go on a diet with her and get together on a regular basis to offer support. The plan worked and the membership grew and grew until today Weight Watchers has helped millions of people lose weight. In fact, without Jean Nidetch, the planet might have actually imploded by now due to all the extra weight it was forced to support.

The reason Weight Watchers has been a success for as long as it has is simple. It is a plan that actually works, and it offers a great deal of support to keep people motivated. Although the specific plans have changed over the years, Weight Watchers offers two plans today that are really quite simple. The most popular one is based on points. Each food is assigned a point value based on a combination of its fiber, calorie, and fat content. Depending on your weight, you're allowed to eat a certain amount of points per day. No one cares whether you use them on three healthy meals a day, or blow them all on a Blizzard from Dairy Queen, as long as you stay within your allotted points.

The second plan is more like a modified Atkins Diet, which allows you to have unlimited portions of certain foods. But unlike Atkins, you're also allowed to have a limited amount of breads and pastas with each meal, as long as they're the right kinds (brown rice, couscous, whole wheat pasta, and so on). Just think of this plan as Atkins "light."

Weight Watchers also offers weekly meetings to provide motivation and support to its members. Each meeting is led by trained personnel who are all well versed in the different plans, and who have the freakish ability to remember a roomful of names as if their brains were fly strips for names. They've also memorized the point value of every food and can recite it as adeptly as men can recite that silly "Who's on first?" routine.

Because Weight Watchers has been around almost as long as vinyl flooring, I decided to give it a try. I went to my first meeting recently and found it to be quite interesting. First, I was greeted by a woman who weighed me on a delightful scale that didn't allow me to see the result. Instead, it was printed out and put into my new handy-dandy booklet, which I was required to bring with me to each weekly meeting and weigh-in.

The meeting lasted a half hour and was chock-full of advice about two-point food finds and how to get through an upcoming holiday. It was also chock-full of advertisements for Weight Watchers products. The leader raved about the company's recipe books, odometers, and magazines. You'd think that her motivation was to help the room lose weight, but I found out later that it was partially due to the fact that she got a percentage of everything sold during her meeting.

All in all, I found that Weight Watchers is a commonsense plan, so I can only find a few negative things to say about it. You are encouraged to attend the weekly meetings, there is a nominal price to pay (I paid about $10 per meeting), and they really do stress exercise. Besides those things, I ended up learning a great deal from Weight Watchers, such as:

1. Slow weight loss really is the healthiest and longest-lasting kind of weight loss.
2. Weight Watchers sells its own line of frozen foods at the markets under the name Smart Ones. The predetermined point value is printed right on the package.

3. Unlike some other diets, Weight Watchers believes it's not important what time of day you eat, as long as you don't go over your assigned number of points.

4. It's much easier to get on a scale when you don't see the number staring back at you.

5. There's a Web site, *www.DWLZ.com*, that lists the point value of most store-bought food items and restaurant menu selections.

6. Orange Chicken is not your friend.

Diets I Could Get My Big 'Ol Behind Behind

The problem with most diets today is that it takes a long time for you to see any results. Since most diets strive to achieve the suggested two pounds a week, you can be on them for months before you get to your goal weight. But it doesn't have to be that way, since there are other ways to lose weight quickly. Sure, some aren't necessarily healthy or approved by the medical profession. Heck, some aren't even legal. But they can all make you slim down faster than you can say "Nicole Richie." Here are some examples:

Have the love of your life walk out on you. Anyone who's ever experienced the pain of a broken heart knows all too well that being dumped is the quickest form of weight loss since childbirth.

Break a law and go to prison. Martha Stewart struggled with her weight for years but never won the battle until she went to camp cupcake and emerged months later looking oh so svelte in her handmade poncho. I guess complete humiliation and institutional cooking can really be "a good thing."

Get a tapeworm. If you've ever seen anyone who's been infected with a tapeworm, you were no doubt amazed at how wonderful that person looked! It's like liposuction in maggot form. I think pharmaceutical companies should be able to sell them at drugstores, right next to the diet pills. They should come with an easy-to-swallow coating and have a string wrapped around one end so that you can remove them like a tampon whenever you reach your goal weight.

Prepackaged airplane food. Instead of buying diet food from Jenny Craig or NutriSystem, think of how much weight you'd lose if you dined exclusively on prepackaged airplane food. Since most airlines are on the verge of bankruptcy, their food is only slightly more appetizing than eating Soylent Green.

Montezuma's revenge in gel-cap form. Each pill would contain all the diarrhea-causing bacteria you'd find in one cup of water south of the border. Sure, you'll be so sick that you'll want to die, but you'll lose weight rapidamente!

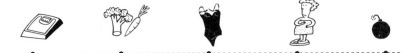

chapter four

the hell you endure
to look better in jeans

For many women, diets are as much a part of the daily regimen as shaving their legs, putting on makeup, and inspecting their chin for that errant stray hair. Granted, there are a handful of lucky women who can eat anything they want without getting fat, but they don't really count. They're considered anomalies of nature, like a two-headed lizard, and besides, nobody really likes them anyway. But real women, those of us who can gain five pounds on a three-day weekend, know a thing or two about diets.

By now, some of you have made the decision to start a diet. Maybe it's due to an upcoming reunion or a vacation that involves wearing clothes that contain spandex. Or maybe it's because you can't even get your fat pants to zip up anymore. Not only have you made the decision to start a diet, but you've decided which diet to start. You've gone over the options and have chosen the plan that no doubt allowed the most amount of snacks and the least amount of exercise.

I know that right now, at the start of your diet, you have tremendous determination to shed those unwanted pounds, and you think that's all you'll need to see your diet through to the end. I'm here to say that you couldn't be more wrong. Remember when you thought that love was all you needed to get through your marriage? Then came the all-weekend sports marathons, the all-night snoring sessions, and the fact that somehow, it became your responsibility to do all the housework and buy every gift for his side of the family even though he has more siblings than the Osmonds. It's then that you realized that it takes a lot more than love to make a relationship work. It also requires a large amount of alcoholic beverages.

In the same manner, it requires much more than determination to get through any diet. The reason? There are so many hidden challenges that go into dieting beyond eating an endless stream of salads. If you are starting a diet, you not only have my sympathy, but also my incredible insight. There are many different factors to consider when starting a diet, all of which can determine the success of its outcome. Let's take a look at what those factors are.

How Low Can You Go?

Every new dieter is faced with the dilemma of picking a goal weight. You have to decide if you want one that's realistic, or a fantasy that can only be achieved by a wired jaw and a liquid diet. When it comes to determining a goal weight, I've found that people depend on two entirely different criteria.

The first is based upon a number on the scale. The dreamy left side of our brain imagines that once we get down to that specific number, our lives will suddenly become wonderful. Our body will be toned, our skin will be bronzed, and our roots will forever be filled in. We will be perpetually lit from behind and our hair will have that carefree windswept look. But the right side of our brain cures the left side's temporary insanity when it calculates just how many pounds we'd actually have to shed in order to attain this fantasy.

For me this fantasy weight is 115. Granted, I haven't weighed that little since I got my first driver's license, and chances are high that I lied about my weight even then. But no matter, that's the weight that I'd always like to return to one day. In hindsight, I don't think I was really content with my body back then. I'm sure that, even at that low weight, I thought I'd look better if I could only manage to drop a few pounds. We women are odd that way and I guarantee that twenty years from now, I'd kill to be the weight that I am right now. We never seem to be content no matter what the scale says, and feel that we'll never be happy unless we return to the weight that we were in utero.

The other criterion when picking a goal weight is to have it be low enough so that we're able to fit into a specific article of clothing that we were able to fit into in the past. We drift off into a state of euphoria as we imagine ourselves finally zipping up that body-hugging slip dress that's been stored in the back of our closet as long as Walt Disney has supposedly been stored in his cryogenic crypt. And like Mr. Disney, we're both equally excited about the coming-out party.

One of the outfits that women most commonly strive to fit into again has got to be their wedding dress. This isn't much of a problem for those who have recently celebrated their paper anniversary, but it can be quite a challenge for those who are nearing their silver. As we stare at the pictures in our wedding albums, we hardly recognize ourselves. We look so thin, and strive to once again attain that model-like figure. We somehow forget the minor detail that it took a month's worth of starvation, a crew of beauticians, and a spleen-crushing corset to attain that hourglass look.

The most famous piece of goal-weight clothing has got to be Oprah Winfrey's skinny jeans. Who can forget when she came out onto the stage of her talk show back in 1988 with her Calvin Klein jeans, her big helmet hair, and her red wagon full of 67 pounds of fat? Although I was happy for Oprah that she was able to achieve her dream, I was also a bit nervous that her oversized head would cause her to tip over headfirst into the fat.

Regardless of which of the two systems you choose to select your goal weight, I think that it's best to think small. Instead of choosing a number that would take months of Diet Coke and Lean Cuisine to achieve, choose one that would take but a week of abstaining from junk food. Once you achieve this goal, pick another number that's just a little higher than the first. Yes, my friend, baby steps is what weight loss is about. Keep the goals easy, keep the numbers realistic, and keep away from a wagon full of fat if you too have big helmet hair.

Setting the Date

Timing in life is everything. Studies show that there are certain times of the day when surgeries are more successful.

There are certain times of the year when driving is safest. And there are certain times of the month when your husband might benefit from wearing a hardhat when he's near you.

Timing is everything when it comes to the day that we start a diet as well. For many of us, this decision could significantly influence the chances of success. So before you decide upon a start date, there are several different factors that you should consider.

The first factor to contemplate is which day of the week to actually begin. Very few people I know start a new diet on a Tuesday or a Thursday. Instead, they prefer to start it on the first workday of the week: Monday. Monday is a great day to delve into a diet considering that most of us spent the majority of the weekend pigging out. Besides, not only is Monday the beginning of the week, but it's also the day of *Monday Night Football*. Because of this, we usually eat alone in the kitchen while our husbands sit in front of the TV talking to the players more than they talked with us the whole entire weekend!

Some dieters take this "starting a diet at the beginning of the week" theory to a whole new level and prefer to start theirs at the beginning of the month. Not only does starting their diet on the first day of the month give them ample time to get motivated, it also makes keeping track of how many days they've been on it a breeze. If it's the tenth day of the month, they've been dieting for ten days. This seems to work well for sleep-deprived parents, busy people with a lot on their mind, and those who need to count on their fingers.

Still others take this theory one step further and refuse to start their diet on anything but the biggest diet day of the whole year: January first. They feel that starting their diet on the first day of the brand-new year gives them a huge psychological advantage over the average dieter. I feel that it's just their way of procrastinating for the longest period of time possible.

Another important factor that must be taken into account when choosing a start date is to choose one that isn't close to an upcoming event or holiday that revolves around food. That may be quite difficult, because there always seems to be some kind of celebration that involves eating. There's always an upcoming birthday party, a family brunch, a office party, or a Saturday night movie date that requires a mandatory bag of bulk candy. So before you pick a start date, look at the calendar and find a day that's not close to Mary's famous onion dip, Lizzy's pavlova, or any food that comes "a la mode."

When setting the date, it's also crucial to factor in your menstrual cycle. As you know, getting a visit from Aunt Flo means eating massive amounts of chocolate and retaining more water than Lake Erie. The most destructive thing that we can do is to struggle through a week of dieting only to find that we've gained three pounds due to premenstrual symptoms. What you *should* do is begin a diet at the beginning of your period, since you're likely to drop a pound or two then anyway.

Just as there are good days to start a diet, there are bad days as well. Here is a list of some of the all-time worst dates to start a diet:

- February 15, when all those unsold heart-shaped boxes of chocolates are on sale.
- Free ice-cream day at Baskin-Robbins.

- Any day that *Goodfellas* is rerun on television.
- Payday, i.e., the day that you have a pocketful of money to burn at that eight-course Moroccan restaurant you've always wanted to try.
- When you're anywhere near Hershey, Pennsylvania.
- Days of predictable high stress, like the start of a new job or when your mother-in-law comes to stay and tells you how to raise your kids . . . I mean, helps you out with your kids.

Fat Tuesday . . . or Wednesday . . . or Thursday

During the past two hundred years, New Orleans has perfected everything from beignets to beans and rice, but nothing has been more perfected than its annual tradition of Mardi Gras. Mardi Gras, which literally means "Fat Tuesday," begins before Lent, the time when Catholics are supposed to abstain from some of their favorite things. Whether it be raindrops on roses or whiskers on kittens (or more likely booze and desserts for those who don't sing high atop mountains), people must give up some of the greatest pleasures in life. But before this abstinence begins, people celebrate Mardi Gras by pigging out on po-boys, munching on muffulettas, and gorging themselves on gumbo.

The "feast or famine" belief system that is seen during Mardi Gras is also utilized whenever one starts a diet. In the same manner as this wise Cajun community, we fill up our bellies with every decadent morsel that we can get our hands on before we too must abstain. We pick out the last crumbs from the empty bag of wafer cookies and lick the container clean of rocky road ice cream. We delve deep into the bowels of our refrigerator in hopes of finding a leftover slice of pizza or a Tupperware container filled with angel hair pasta. Yes, before we start any new diet, we transform into Magellan exploring our fridge for any undiscovered treasures.

This "feast before the famine" tradition is one that's very commonly found in nature. Any animal that hibernates must eat a great quantity of food before it settles in for the winter. If gorging oneself on nuts and berries works for bears and squirrels, it should work well enough for me. After all, we're all God's creatures great and small, and the greater we are, the more nuts and berries, and angel hair pasta, we need to eat before starting our own self-inflicted famine.

Sure, we could just toss all these fatty leftovers into the trash instead of into our mouths. That would indeed be a much smarter thing to do. But somehow eating ourselves into oblivion before we start a diet may just provide us with the psychological advantage we need to lose weight. The same theory has been applied to other addictions, like cigarette smoking. I remember that my Uncle Morris tried to quit by going to the Schick Center years ago and smoking a whole pack of cigarettes in under two hours. You'd think he would have been disgusted, but he loved the experience and thought of it as his version of a spa day. Nonetheless, the idea of having your own Fat Tuesday, or Fat whatever day of the week you choose, may just make you so sick and disgusted with yourself that you actually will look forward to beginning your diet.

Once you're done with this spring cleaning of your refrigerator, you need to make sure that there aren't any high-calorie temptations left lying around to call to you during a craving binge. Sure, you may not see anything left on the shelves, but there are several hidden nooks and crannies that you'll need to explore before you fill the shelves full of cottage cheese and carrot sticks:

1. Make sure that you look deep in the right- and left-hand back corners of the lower shelf. There always seems to be a lone pudding cup or an open container of sour cream, which houses the leftover onion dip.

2. Check out the butter compartment. If your husband is like mine and only ventures into the fridge to grab a quick beer, the butter compartment is an excellent place to hide your secret stash. Not only can it conceal your bite-sized chocolates, but it's the perfect place to store any love letters from past boyfriends and receipts from your last shopping spree.

3. Explore the cheese drawer. Make sure you get rid of the last nibble of that decadent Maytag cheese wedge and the addicting garlic-and-herb spread that haunts you late at night.

Now that you've picked a start date, and cleaned out your refrigerator so well that you can see your reflection in the meat drawer, you've completed each and every pre-diet task. Now you're ready to jump headfirst into the depths of diethood. But before you do, take a deep breath, hold your nose, and pray that the water won't be so shocking that it causes cardiac arrest.

I'm So Hungry I Could Eat My Hair.
Hell, I Could Eat Your Hair.

Not long after eating your first diet meal, you get hit with hunger pains. This may happen several hours after breakfast, or, if you're anything like me, immediately after you clean up the breakfast dishes. It's at this point that you're hit with one of the hardest parts about going on a diet: being hungry. In fact, if it weren't for the damn hunger thing, most diets would be a relative breeze to follow.

Now, you may be saying to yourself, "[Insert name here], isn't it actually called a hunger *pang* instead of a pain?" Well, [insert name here], you may be correct. I've seen it used both ways, but I prefer to call it a hunger *pain*. The reason for this is simple. It hurts. And if something hurts, I try to get rid of the pain as soon as possible. If I have a headache, I reach for Tylenol. If I have a backache, I reach for a heating pad. And if I have a hunger pain, I reach for chocolate chip banana bread. So you can understand that when I'm on a diet and denied access to my chocolate chip banana bread, I am not a happy camper.

The reason for these agonizing internal pains is that when a stomach is empty, it contracts due to lack of food and low blood sugar. Interestingly enough, I learned that if you're a younger person, your hunger pains tend to be stronger than they would be if you were older, due to your better gastrointestinal muscle tone. I guess there are definite advantages to growing older after all.

The way I see it, hunger pains are quite similar to labor pains. In both instances, the contractions become more and more intense as the minutes goes by, and in both instances, all you want to do is yell at your spouse. But unlike labor pains, which are easily cured by simply pushing out a kid, hunger pains can linger for days or even months!

At first you do what every diligent dieter would do to appease them. You drink water like your diet book suggests. And for a while, it does manage to take the edge off. But after you've had enough water to fill the grotto at the Playboy mansion, you resort to Plan B. You try to placate your stomach by feeding it tiny tidbits of diet food. Maybe a couple of celery stalks, or, if you're on Atkins, a pork butt. Again, it seems to work for a while, but soon the hunger pains return, and this time, they've come back with a vengeance! They strike relentlessly with the force of the dark side and suddenly, you're out of control. You look at a piece of Wonder bread as if you were Mike Tyson and it was Evander Holyfield's ear. In fact, you're so hungry that you crave foods that you never thought you could stomach before. After decades of confusion, it suddenly becomes clear how the passengers from that book *Alive* could be so hungry they'd resort to cannibalism.

It's at this point that your diet could easily come to a screeching halt. You see that open box of vanilla wafers in the front of the cabinet and you could grab them as easily as Jude Law could grab a nanny. But you don't. You're a good little dieter and you are strong. You find the inner strength to work through the pain, and you get your second wind. Let's just hope that in twenty minutes, when the next contraction sets in, you can be just as strong. Until then, if you want to feel better, go ahead and yell at your spouse. Chances are that you picked up his dirty underwear from the bathroom floor again this morning, so you're definitely entitled.

Hell on Meals

I'm not telling you anything new when I say that diet food sucks. You know this just as well as I do and are fully aware that it's bland, dull, and tasteless diet cuisine that makes dieting oh so difficult. You wake up in the morning craving your usual cup of coffee and a side of cinnamon roll, but instead have to force-feed your face an egg-white omelet with sautéed spinach. You leave the table with your stomach feeling hungry, your willpower feeling challenged, and your teeth feeling gritty from all that spinach. A few hours later when lunchtime rolls around, you want a yummy meatloaf sandwich with seasoned curly fries from the local diner (otherwise known as "the usual"). But once again, you deny yourself what you crave and eat a Beef & Broccoli Lean Cuisine that, to me, has all the taste of a salt lick.

Yes, it seems that having to eat diet food is an enormous obstacle when it comes to successful dieting. Gone are the days when you gorge yourself on gluttonous foods full of carbs, sugar, and fat. All that remains to eat now are low-calorie versions of your favorite fattening foods, such as fat-free cheese, whose only similarity to the original is that it has the ability to cause constipation.

Who knows? Maybe I'm just a bit more sensitive to diet food than the average dieter is. To be honest, I'm a bit of a food snob. I consider myself a good cook and spend more time with the chefs on the Food Network than I do with some members of my own family. I know all of *Sara's Secrets*, and I've kicked many a meal up a notch with Emeril. I buy tomato sauce made from San Marziano tomatoes, use sea salt in all of my cooking, and have dined in restaurants that were given more stars than Patton.

Then there are the people who are more like my husband and don't care much about food labels. His idea of the perfect meal is a fried bologna sandwich, a cold hot dog pulled straight from the package, and a side of anything that's smothered in gravy. My husband couldn't tell you the difference between Wesson oil and truffle oil if his life depended on it.

I have a theory about dieting. I believe that you'll have more success on a diet if you're a person like my husband; someone who has very few food preferences. But if you're a foodie like me, you'll need these simple tips to help the diet food go down:

1. Subscribe to the Food Network on your cable or satellite system. There are several cooking shows that will teach you how to make delicious low-calorie or low-carb meals.

2. Add fresh herbs to your food whenever you can. A sprinkle of fresh thyme can make even boiled tofu taste good (well, okay, maybe not good, but better).

3. If your diet allows, use a lot of hot sauce on your meals. Not only will this give your food an added kick, it should also singe away the majority of your taste buds, making future diet food more palatable.

4. Hold your nose while you eat diet food. It works with a kid taking his medicine, and it'll work for that low-carb bread that has all the taste of a wad of gristle.

5. Eat by candlelight. Sure, it won't make your food taste any better, but it will sure make it look a whole lot less disgusting.

Chef Boy, Are You Tired from Doing All of This Cooking?

If there's ever a time when you need to know your way around a kitchen, it's when you're on a diet. Suddenly, cooking a meal requires a lot more time and effort than it did in the past, when all you had to do to prepare a sumptuous feast was open up a can of bean dip and pour it over a plateful of tortilla chips. Yes, to fix a meal these days, you'll need kitchen gadgets beyond your basic can opener.

Now that you're eating fresh, healthy foods, you'll need instruments to prepare them, like sharp knives, electric juicers, and dangerous food processors that can turn your hand into that of your old shop teacher with just the push of a button. And, in order to cook these meals, you'll need more than just your microwave. You'll need broiler pans, vegetable steamers, and indoor grills. Don't be surprised if your husband suspects that you're having affair with some new guy you're always seeing: Williams-Sonoma.

If you're into more exotic cuisine, like French or Japanese, you may need to take this even one step further. In order to prepare some of these specialized meals, you may want tools such as a mandoline, a sieve, a microplane, and a Silpat. If you thought finding your G-spot was a challenge, wait till you have to track down some of these cooking oddities.

In addition to the many extra kitchen tools that you'll need to create diet fare, there are also additional trips to the supermarket. Instead of buying your meals at taco stands and fast-food joints, you'll now have to venture into unfamiliar territory such as farmers' markets and produce sections. That's because cooking healthy requires using fresh ingredients, like fruits and vegetables, that tend to spoil faster than

> **❝**I never did much cooking before I went on the Zone, but now I'm in the kitchen all the time cutting and dicing fresh vegetables. I think the majority of the weight I lost is due to the fact that I've cut my fingers so many times, I'm down a few pints of blood.**❞**
>
> —Katie

a kid from Beverly Hills. Fruits quickly overripen and get mushy. Vegetables get coated with a slimy substance that resembles the stuff that covers a newborn baby. Because of this, you'll have to replace these items far more often than their frozen or canned versions. Yes, dieting would certainly be a lot easier if Mother Nature would just sprinkle some preservatives over her farm-fresh goodies.

When I diet, I find going to all this trouble of food preparation extremely frustrating. I detest spending more time fixing a meal than I do eating it. And cleaning up from all that cooking is also a time-consuming job. No longer does tidying up mean tossing a fast-food wrapper in the trash. From here on in it requires soaking, scrubbing, and constant dishpan hands. When you're on a diet, every meal becomes its own little Thanksgiving dinner.

If your household is anything like mine, mealtimes are already a nightmare. There are so many fussy mouths to feed that I have to prepare three separate meals. My husband is a meat-and-potatoes guy who refuses to eat any vegetables besides onion rings, and my six-year-old is only willing to eat food that is yellow (it used to be white, so at least we're working up the color chart). When I throw in the additional challenge of preparing a low-calorie, healthy meal for myself, I feel as if I'm a short-order cook. I guess I could just prepare one low-calorie, healthy meal that my whole family could enjoy, but that's one of those fantasies that's never as good in reality, like when you took your two-year-old to the art museum because you thought he'd appreciate culture, when in fact, it only inspired him to draw a mural of his own from the goodies found in his diapers.

If you're really having a hard time in the kitchen, here are some basic staples that you should keep stocked in your fridge and pantry to make the chore of cooking healthy a whole lot easier:

1. **Bagged lettuce.** It's usually precut and prewashed. The only thing that would make it easier is if it were pre-dressed.

2. **Frozen fruit and veggies.** Sure, they may not be as healthy as fresh, but they certainly are a whole lot easier. They're also one step above canned in terms of taste and health benefits.

3. **Preminced garlic.** I find that garlic that's already cut and bottled tastes just as good as fresh and doesn't leave any of that smelly garlic scent on your fingers that you can never seem to get rid of no matter how many times you wash your hands.

4. **Precut chopped onion.** Not only will this save you time, it'll also save you a fortune in bandages!

5. **Precut carrots and celery.** They're great in your cooking, and a great handy snack.

6. **Precooked, presliced chicken breast, which you'll find in the deli meat section.** Having this stuff around is so much easier than cooking the chicken yourself and cutting it up. It's more expensive, but it's a huge timesaver.

7. **Light sauces.** Check the deli section near the refriger-
   ated pastas for low-cal and low-fat sauces.
8. **Whole wheat tortillas.** These make a great substitute
   for bread. They're high-fiber and low-calorie and-carb,
   and you can use them to make great fast burritos.
9. **Boiled eggs.** Use the egg whites to toss into a salad, or
   make them into an egg-white salad (just like regular
   egg salad but far less caloric).
10. **Non-cream soups.** They're filling and easy to make.
11. **Whole-grain cereal.** Not only is this good for breakfast,
    but it's also a good substitute when you have a craving
    to down a bag of potato chips. If you munch on whole-
    grain flakes, it's harder to pig out.

Serving Size Matters

Now that you're learning how to prepare your own healthy,
low-calorie meals, you need to know how much food to
actually put on your plate. This can be quite a challenge
for those of us who haven't eaten a proper serving size since
we were weaned off the bottle. As you know, human beings
have evolved substantially over the last several million years
and are still undergoing many physiological transformations
today. For instance, we no longer need our appendix because
we don't graze on grass, and we're no longer covered with
thick body hair, because we have Old Navy fleece pullovers
to help keep us warm. But the most significant change that's
taken place in our bodies is the one that occurred about fifty
years ago, when we somehow lost our ability to know what
a serving size looks like.

If you look back at the 1950s, you'll realize that an amazing number of discoveries took place during that time period. It marked the beginning of space travel, the invention of the polio vaccine, and the biggest creation of them all, the TV dinner. Back in the '50s, people were satisfied with a TV dinner that contained a couple of slices of turkey, a small scoop of peas, and a dollop of mashed potatoes. Those portions seem more like appetizers by today's standards, considering that our version of this dining classic is the Hungry-Man dinner, which weighs in at over a pound of food. Somehow between then and now, the average serving size has spun out of control. Back in 1957, the typical fast-food burger had 210 calories. Today, it has a whopping 618 calories!

With many diet plans, you have to adhere to strict portions. Some diets spell out exactly how much food you can eat. They instruct you to have a 6-ounce serving of this or 40 grams of that. Measuring out these quantities may not be such a problem for you if you weigh cocaine for a living, but for most of us average folk, the task can be rather daunting. In addition to all of the kitchen gadgets you need to prepare your meal, you'll now need the additional help of a measuring cup, a kitchen scale, and a postage meter to figure out just how many green beans to put on your plate.

I find this part of a diet rather difficult. I consider myself a smart person (barring those times I do really stupid things like remove sap on my car hood with nail polish remover), so it frustrates me to no end when I can't figure out how much London broil to eat. I've been told that a serving size of meat is about the size of a credit card, but how thick should it be? It can't be the width of a credit card because that would be too cruel.

Since you're just starting out on your diet, don't be surprised if you're having trouble figuring out portion size too. If you are, you may want to consider going on a diet like Jenny Craig or NutriSystem, which takes all the guesswork out for you. Their prepackaged meals have just the right amount of food to make your diet effective. Some diets, like Atkins, require no portion size at all. In fact, you can eat a whole cow in one sitting and still adhere to the diet (of course you'll have to milk the cow first, because dairy isn't allowed).

Sometimes diets use code words to determine just how much food you can eat. Diets like Weight Watchers use points to measure their meals. Others like Sugar Busters! use numbers from a glycemic index. But I find the most confusing unit of measure to be what they call "net carbs." I know that a net carb has something to do with how many carbohydrates a certain food has, minus the fiber or fat or something else it contains, but it's just one of those things that I'll never *fully* understand, like how a plane flies or what's going on with Donald Trump's hair.

Once you determine what a serving size is (for help see page 46), then comes the even harder part to manage: being satisfied with it. Yes, it's hard leaving the table feeling full when you've eaten just a fraction of the amount of food that you used to eat. If you're having trouble filling up on 1950s-size portions, here are a few ideas that may help you be satisfied:

1. Put your food on small plates. Your food will be smushed together and give the illusion that you're actually eating more than you are. Optical illusions are really quite effective, and in fact are responsible for the success of Salvador Dali.

2. If your diet allows, use a lot of fillers when preparing your meals. Fill a sandwich with loads of lettuce and veggies. Add grated zucchini, carrots, squash, or other vegetables to your meatloaf. This is the system that the Chinese have followed for centuries, which explains why every takeout container is half full of those water chestnuts that no one ever seems to eat.

3. Go ahead, lick the bowl. If you're only allowed two tablespoons of tomato sauce on your pasta, you're entitled to every last drop. In fact, if a drop falls onto your blouse, you have permission to lick up that too.

4. Cut up your food into small bites so that it'll last longer. It's also a good idea to use smaller utensils. Substitute a teaspoon for a soup spoon when eating cereal and soups to give yourself more bites of food.

5. In addition to using a fork and a knife at every meal, you should also make use of a magnifying glass. It's guaranteed to supersize any meal.

Too Much Math

If you had a hard time back in school figuring out just how fast a train would get to the station if it was going east at 122 mph on the first Tuesday of the month when the moon was in the gibbous stage, then wait until you try to figure out the calorie, carbohydrate, or point count of all of your food every time you sit down to eat. Suddenly, every meal becomes its own little SAT.

Take something as simple as a sandwich. In days past you would fix yourself one of these delicious devils without thinking twice. You'd layer on the mayonnaise, the meat and cheese, a few slices of lettuce and tomato, and if you really felt wild, you'd add a few potato chips for some extra crunch. But now, calculating the calorie count of that simple pleasure in life would involve NASA's ground control and that guy they wrote *A Beautiful Mind* about.

Sure, you may have a reference book that contains the calorie count of every food from apples to zucchini so you can calculate each individual sandwich item, but figuring that out would take longer than it would to digest the sandwich. Luckily, you can take advantage of living in the Internet age and can check out Web sites that contain charts of your favorite foods. They even have some that list items at your favorite restaurants. Individual diet programs like Weight Watchers usually have their own sites, which offer help for your specific diet.

Those on a low-carb diet can visit several Web sites that list the carbohydrate count of foods. If you're on the Atkins diet, you know that you're restricted to eating only 20 grams of carbohydrates each day. That's why it's so crucial to keep track of every itty-bitty morsel of food that you eat. You don't want to blow a day's worth of dieting by taking a bite of a lousy apple.

As you can see, it's tedious but important to be aware of everything you eat, whether it be in the form of a calorie, a carb, or a point. Look at it this way—by doing this, you'll not only get a smaller body, but all that addition may even sharpen your mind enough that you can once and for all figure out just what time that damn train gets to the station.

Withdrawals

As we've previously discussed in this book, I believe that you can actually become addicted to food. I don't care if the medical community agrees with me or not. What do they know anyway? They used to believe that eating chocolate caused acne. If that were true, there'd be a lot of schoolkids walking around with bad skin, now wouldn't there? Maybe I need a better example. Okay, they used to believe that the sun's rays would cause premature aging. If that were true, there'd be a whole lot of people in Southern California getting plastic surgery . . . Well, maybe we should just move on.

I think you can become addicted to food, and can therefore go into withdrawal when you go on a diet and have to abstain from a certain food. What is a diet, really, if not for a time when you're forced to continually deny yourself the foods that you crave? Meal after meal, snack after snack, you deprive your body of the sugar, the carbs, and the fat that it so desperately "needs" in order to make it through an average day.

I know firsthand the effect on my body when I deprive it of its minimum daily requirement of sweets, and I'm telling you, it ain't pretty! When a craving hits, I look through my cupboards searching for a fix with the intensity of an Amber Alert. Anything will do. A forgotten piece of candy corn from Halloween. A leftover chocolate egg from Easter. Then finally, I find something! Behind the coffee mugs and the expired vitamins is an old Viactiv chocolate calcium chew. Elated, I blow off the dust and stray dog hair from the wrapper, pop the chew in my mouth, and savor every last morsel of its goodness as I feel the sugar slowly enter my blood stream! Ahhhhh!

> **"**I had an interview lined up to work as a tour guide for Universal Studios. I'd heard they liked their guides to be thin so I starved myself for a week. I ended up quitting the diet and passing on the interview altogether. I figured if I had to go through all that hell to be skinny, I'd rather pursue my real dream of being an actress not just a stupid tour guide.**"**
>
> —Lisa

If you're an addict too, then prepare to go through a variety of withdrawal symptoms when you start your diet, none of which will be pretty. I've compiled a list of what you can expect to endure when you go cold turkey. I know that the symptoms I've listed below are those that usually describe the symptoms of withdrawal from illicit drugs, but as you can see, addiction is addiction whether it's to cocaine or coconut cupcakes.

Full-body shakes: Whenever you deny your body its regular food supply, you can expect to feel like a martini being shaken, not stirred.

Headaches: A very common sign of withdrawal is a headache. When you cut your brain off from its fuel supply, namely glucose and sucrose or any other technical name for sugar, it's not a happy cranium.

Lack of focus: One very common complaint among dieters is their inability to concentrate. For the first time in your life, you might miss your usual off ramp and not even notice until you're halfway through Texas. Although the medical community suggests this condition is caused by low blood sugar, I believe it's due to the fact that 98 percent of your mental capacity is busy fantasizing about being on death row so you could have one great meal without worrying that you'll put on weight the next day.

You'll go to extreme measures to get a fix: Just as driving in rush-hour traffic makes you suddenly understand road rage, being on a diet makes you suddenly understand why drug addicts will steal from family and friends in order to get a fix. I too have done things that I'm ashamed of, like eating a customer's leftover pizza when I was a waitress.

Obsession: Before you restricted your daily caloric intake, you were a sane, rational person. Now you're more like a teenage boy with a one-track mind. But instead of being obsessed with girls, you're obsessed with Girl Scout Cookies.

Personality disorders: Not only can a diet change your waist-line, it can also change your personality. No matter which diet you choose, you can experience tremendous mood swings. Well, truthfully, there really isn't much swinging involved since you pretty much stay in the "irritable cranky bitch" position for the duration.

How Long Until I Can Eat?

Do you remember those boring classes back in school when you'd spend the whole time just watching the clock tick? For me, the most boring of them all was my Spanish class, taught by Miss Falcinella. Miss Falcinella was 185 years old and moved with the speed of gridlock traffic. Those exciting days of yesteryear will return to you now that you're on a diet, because all you do all day is watch the clock, waiting endlessly for your next meal. It seems that once you start a diet, life becomes one endless Spanish class.

The reason that you live for your next meal is simple. Your single piece of whole-wheat bread with half a grapefruit didn't fill you up the same way those four McGriddles did in the past. So you eagerly await lunch as if it were a half-off sale at Bloomingdale's. Chances are high that you're starved an hour later and can't make it until the hands strike noon to eat. So you decide to have an early lunch, say around 10:15 or so, and have your afternoon snack by 1:00. By 4:00 you've already had your dinner, so you're done eating for the day and your mail hasn't even been delivered yet.

Some of you may have a harder time waiting to eat than others. If you're anything like me, you have a tendency to snack throughout the day. You also have a tendency to make a mental to-do list while having sex, but let's stick to the issue at hand. I'm used to eating several small meals throughout the day. (Actually, is sixty-five still considered "several"? I'm never quite sure how that works.) So when I'm limited to eating only three squares a day with a pity snack thrown in for good measure, I have a hard time coping. It'd be like telling a cow not to graze in a field all day. Now that's a diet guaranteed to cause mad cow disease!

Even though eating only three meals a day sounds barbaric, there is one good thing that comes out of it. You have a lot more free time in your day since you don't have to spend so much time waiting in long lines at drive-throughs, washing sink loads of dirty dishes, and struggling to open "easy open" lids that are never really easy to open at all. I estimate that by eating only three times a day, you'll have about thirty-five extra minutes to do with as you please. Here are some ideas on how you can fill your newfound free time.

1. Spend more time with your kids. (Except of course if they're going through that terrible whiny stage that finally ends when they're...hmmm, does it actually ever end? If this is the case, just go to the Gap instead.)
2. Volunteer at an old-age home. Not only will you be bringing joy to others, but you'll leave feeling grateful that your metabolism really isn't as slow as it could be.
3. Work part-time at a meatpacking plant. The nausea you'll feel should make it a breeze to make it to your next meal.
4. Exercise. (Yeah, right.)

I imagine that over time, one could get used to eating just three meals a day. I hear the French people do it, and look at what amazing figures they have. And when they do eat, it's nothing but fattening croissants, buttery pastries, and heavy cream sauces. Granted, the French don't actually eat much of that food since they spend most of their lunch hour drinking wine and smoking, but it's a system that works quite well for them nonetheless.

Dieting in Margarita Ville

I'm a firm believer that if you're going to go on a diet, it's best to do it drunk. Having an alcoholic beverage takes the edge off of hunger pains, or maybe it just makes you care about them a whole lot less. It also makes the days go by faster since booze tends to make you walk around in a thick haze that time cannot permeate. The problem with being loopy all day when you're dieting is that certain diets restrict the consumption of alcohol, and if you're on one of those, then dieting is going to suck bigtime.

Even though I don't like having to give up my evening cocktail, I do understand the logic behind restricting this kind of beverage. To begin with, alcohol is loaded with sugar. It's basically a DoveBar in a shot glass. And as you know, when there's sugar, calories are not too far behind. Second, when you're schnookered, you may not have the same degree of will-power that you had before, and may not be able to stop your hand from grabbing that fistful of smoked almonds. There-fore, if you're the kind of person who loves to nurse a glass of wine or down a couple of stiff apple martinis, you should steer clear of diets that kiss Kahlúa and cream goodbye.

If you do enjoy a glass of wine at the end of a day, you should avoid going on diets like South Beach (you can't have any alcohol during the first two weeks) and Somersizing (actually, on Somersizing you're allowed to cook with wine, so you can relax at the end of a day with a tall glass of sauce). Instead, you should consider Sugar Busters! or a similar diet. Sugar Busters! allows you to have a glass of wine as long as you drink it on a full stomach. Weight Watchers too allows alcoholic beverages, as long as you stay within your point limit. And, although Atkins doesn't allow wine or sweet drinks, it does allow certain kinds of hard liquor, such as vodka and gin, to wash down all that bacon fat.

If you simply enjoy the taste of beer but don't care so much about the alcohol, you may want to consider the bevy of non-alcoholic beverages to choose from at your local supermarket or liquor store. Personally, I never quite understood the point of drinking nonalcoholic beer. I guess it's for people who don't like to get drunk but do like to pee a lot.

So remember, if you like to drink and you're on a diet that restricts alcohol, adhering to that diet may be quite a difficult task. If a diet doesn't allow one to eat or drink, I for one am certainly not going to be merry.

Night Terrors

Not only is dieting a tremendous struggle to endure during the day; it can be a tremendous struggle to endure during the night as well. For one thing, it's hard to fall asleep when every molecule of your being is urging you to go to the kitchen and eat something dipped in ranch dressing. For another, it's impossible to drift off to la-la land with the sound of your stomach growling like a dying cat all night. For anyone who doesn't know, a growling stomach is even more annoying than a snoring husband, and believe me, I know far too well just how annoying the latter can be.

Even though it's difficult to fall asleep, many diet gurus believe that going to bed hungry is the right way to lose weight. They say it's as if your body is telling you that yes, you did eat fewer calories during the day than you burned off, and that you're going to wake up in the morning being thinner than you were the day before. Their theory is that you should eat like a king at breakfast, a prince at lunch, and a pauper at dinner. My theory is that if you eat this way, you'll be the town idiot because you'll be sleep-deprived and loopy from being up all night.

But there are other people who don't agree with this caste-system-like way of eating. Diets like Weight Watchers don't have any specific rules that dictate what time of the day you should consume your food. For all they care, you could starve yourself during the day and then scarf down 20 points' worth of Milano cookies at bedtime, and they'd be perfectly okay with it (your partner may not be so keen on the idea since the bed will be full of crumbs, but if he snores all night long, who is he to make demands?).

I guess if I were really a thorough author, I would spend two weeks eating a low-calorie diet early on in the day, and then eat the exact same diet for the next two weeks, but late in the evening. Then I could compare and contrast the weight-loss difference between those two weeks and let you know precisely which method works best. But to tell you the truth, that'd be an awful lot of work for me to do when I know full well that this book will never win a Pulitzer.

Instead, I'll simply pass on some dieting words of wisdom. First, I suggest that you find that perfect time of the evening to eat your last meal of the day—a time that's not so early that you're tempted to binge later on or fall asleep hungry with visions of sugarplums dancing in your head. Second, if your diet allows, you could have a small snack just before retiring for the day. A glass of milk would be a good idea because it's a natural sleep inducer. So is turkey for that matter, because it contains a chemical called tryptophan that should lull you right off to sleep. In fact, why don't you have a big glass of turkey milk just before bed? Wait, do turkeys actually have milk? Never mind—that's more research for me to do, and I think we both know where I stand on that. Finally, you can try counting sheep, but that doesn't always work. Being as hungry as you are, it doesn't take long before those adorable barnyard creatures transform themselves into succulent chops with a rosemary crust and a side of mint jelly.

No matter what you decide to eat or not to eat before going to bed, falling asleep when you're on a diet can be a quite a struggle indeed. Even if you do finally manage to drift off to dreamland, it can be hard to stay there. I find that I'm constantly up and down all night, although now that I think about it, it may have less to do with the diet and more to do with the construction noise going on deep within my husband's nostrils. I tell you, the only thing that sucks more than sleeping on a diet is sleeping with a snorer. Hey, I think I just figured out the topic of my next book!

Constant Cravings

One of the worst, and I mean worst parts about going on a diet are the cravings. When you think of cravings you conjure up images of a pregnant woman gobbling down vats of pickles and ice cream. But the cravings of a pregnant woman pale in comparison to those of a dieter. Sure, a pregnant woman's needs are motivated by her innate desire to keep her unborn child healthy, but a dieter's needs are motivated by her desire to look sensational in a bias-cut dress. Now that, my friend, is a strong motivation!

During the first few days of starting a new diet, the cravings are always the most intense. Hell, who am I kidding? The cravings are always intense, no matter what stage of the diet you're on. It's just that as time goes by, you're supposed to be able to deal with them better, which is a skill that I have yet to master. I guess it's all a case of mind over matter, and you simply have to build up enough mental strength to endure it, like those guys who can walk over hot coals without screaming, or those wives who can keep their mouths shut when their husbands forget to change the empty roll of toilet paper for the millionth time.

Fighting off a craving involves more mental strength than bending a spoon with your mind. In fact, when a craving hits, I believe that you experience a kind of temporary insanity. I swear that when I put my daughter's leftover ice-cream birthday cake in the freezer, it actually called my name. I suddenly became a schizophrenic and was able to hear voices from deep inside my Kenmore telling me to grab a fork and dive right in. Yes, I had become Squeaky Fromme and the cake had all the mind-controlling powers of Charles Manson.

It was at this point that I had to conjure up every ounce of willpower that I had left in my being. I knew that if I gave in to the cake's wishes and ate up all those succulent purple frozen roses, my diet would be blown for good. Each petal full of goodness contains a day's worth of calories, and I'm talking about a busy day that includes a half hour on the treadmill and volunteering at my kid's school on "make a volcano" day.

If you're being tempted by a highly caloric temptation and your willpower is weaker than the reception on your stolen HBO, try using one of the following techniques to give yourself added strength:

- Destroy the item of temptation. Pour salt all over it and then throw it away. I mention the salt part because I know that if you skip that step, you'll be tempted to eat it right out of the trashcan. Go ahead and deny it. We both know the truth.

- Wait it out. Tell yourself that if you still want it in thirty minutes, you can have it then. Chances are that after thirty minutes, the craving will pass, or someone else will have eaten the tempting morsel first.
- Turn on one of those graphic surgery programs where they show a woman getting a 200-pound tumor removed. This should kill your appetite immediately.

A Food Chart for Real Food

Although there are ample books and Web sites that list the calorie count of foods, there is one inherent problem. The foods that they list are foods like one large apple, half a cup of rice, and a dozen asparagus spears. If someone actually ate foods like these, they wouldn't have a weight problem to begin with. I propose that someone publish a calorie-count book and a matching Web site that's composed of food that people with a weight problem actually consume. Foods such as these:

- A big bowl of sugary cereal with cream
- A bag of pretzels dipped in frosting
- A peanut butter and banana sandwich on white bread
- A generous slice of mayonnaise cake
- A slice of sausage pizza dipped in ranch dressing
- A shot of Cheez Whiz squirted directly into your mouth
- A mouthful of canned whipped cream squirted directly into your mouth

- A bowl of chocolate ice cream with warm peanut butter added
- A BLT sandwich with extra B and none of that annoying L&T

If a calorie book like this one existed, we heavy people would know exactly how many fat grams, carbs, and calories are in the foods that we *actually* eat, making it quite clear how we got into this mess in the first place.

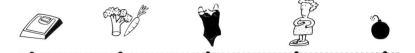

chapter five

no pain, no gain . . .
no thank you!

I'm not really into pain, thank you very much, and I try to
avoid it at all costs. I'm a firm believer in having an epidural
during deliveries, having Novocain when getting a cavity
filled, and turning the channel whenever I land on an old
episode of *The Brady Bunch* in which Jan is going to sing.
So as you can see, I certainly don't go out of my way to seek
out the pain of exercise three times a week for an hour at
a pop. I don't find anything fun about being out of breath
and sweaty unless, of course it involves a man and a squeeze
container of chocolate syrup. In fact, I usually try to avoid
exercise at all cost. I take the elevator instead of the stairs. I
drive to the corner market instead of walk. And my idea of a
good warmup is reheating my sweet roll until the icing gets
all melty and gooey.

But even though I hate to exercise, I force myself to do
it from time to time, like when I'm being chased by my
neighbor's devil dog, and when I decide to go on a diet. I'm

no fool, and I know that exercise will help me lose unwanted pounds by burning additional calories and speeding up my sluggish metabolism all day long. So whenever I decide to go through the hell of a diet, I also force myself to go through the hell of putting on my tight sports bra and getting some exercise (although sometimes, just putting on that damn sports bra turns out to be exercise enough).

The reason that we modern-day *Homo sapiens* have to go out and seek exercise is that we live in an era that's devoid of any need to actually do any. The vast majority of us no longer have to hike miles to the river for water. We don't have to help our neighbor build a barn. And we no longer walk three miles in the snow, uphill both ways, to get to school the way our grandfathers did back when cities must have been really poorly designed. Today we sit in our cars commuting to the office, sit behind our desks all day at work, and sit in our recliners at night watching television. Thanks to modern-day miracles, there's no need to move a muscle. Interoffice e-mail allows us to distribute memos without moving a muscle, and remote controls allow us to change channels without getting our butts up off the couch. Because of our lethargic lifestyle, we really have to go out and seek exercise if we want to incorporate it into our daily lives.

Nonetheless, we know that exercise is something we must do in order to keep ourselves healthy and make our diet more efficient. So if you decide to incorporate exercise into your weight loss plan, here are the good, the bad, and the ugly facts you should know before you go out and get physical (unless it's the kind of physical that you need the man and chocolate syrup for, in which case, you need a different kind of book!).

Don't Be Fooled

Ignorance is bliss for many things in life (like knowing just how many millions of dust mites live in your pillow), but ignorance is not a very useful a tool when it comes to dieting. In fact, naiveté can be the death of any diet and exercise program, especially for those who think that they can easily work off the calories of a croissant simply by doing a few crunches. When it comes to the success of your weight-loss program, you should keep your eyes open and your mouth closed, particularly when it comes anywhere near that flaky French breakfast treat.

I fell victim to this ignorance once myself. I naively thought that if I worked out hard enough in the morning, I could more or less eat whatever I wanted during the day. I thought that a good half-hour run would easily make up for that four-cheese pizza when in reality, it barely covered even *one* of the cheeses. I was uneducated about how many calories exercise truly burns off and ended up getting angry that I had killed myself working out, and still hadn't lost the weight I had hoped to lose.

Since you may be going through the hell of a diet right now, I don't want you to fall victim to the same kind of misconception that I did. The truth is that, while exercise is wonderful for your health, it may not be as wonderful as you thought it was in terms of burning calories. Although there are some exceptions, like running up a hill or taking an advanced spinning class, most forms of exercise only burn off a fraction of the calories they feel like they do for the agony you endure to actually do them. For instance, did you know that if you walked for half an hour, you would barely burn up the calories in a lousy slice of pizza? If you sweated through a moderate bike ride for half an hour, you would hardly burn up the calories in a dry whole-wheat bagel. In fact, even if you indulged in fifteen minutes of vigorous sex, you could only rationalize eating a tomato.

In these examples, the calorie count of the foods is *equal* to the calories you burn off from the exercises. As you know, when you diet, the goal is to eat less than you actually burn off. Therefore, you couldn't have the slice of pizza unless you walked more than half an hour. You'd only be able to eat half the bagel if you wanted your bike ride to count. And, in order to lose weight by having vigorous sex, you'd have to mention the words "mother" and "tampon" from time to time to slow him down.

I don't mean to discourage anyone from exercising; I only wish to educate. I want you to know that if you're one of the many people who believe you'll whittle away the pounds by swimming a few laps in a pool, be warned. If you're not careful, your naiveté can actually cause you to gain weight. We women are funny creatures—if we gain weight even though we're exercising, we rationalize it by telling ourselves that we must have gained muscle, which, as we know from any "Body by Jake" infomercial, weighs more than fat.

While we're on the subject of ignorance regarding exercise, you should also know that many of the so-called energy bars that people gobble up while working out can have just as many calories as a candy bar. Even those neon-colored sports drinks can be a hidden danger. Sure, they replenish things like electrolytes, but if abused, they'll also replenish things like back fat burned off during your two-hour step class.

If you want to improve your mind in the hopes of improving your body, then log on to any number of computer Web sites that specify exactly how many calories you burn off while doing a certain activity. My personal favorite is *www.caloriesperhour.com.* These cyberlists can be quite detailed and specific, so there is no guesswork involved. Some even give you information about how many calories you burn off while doing nonexercise activities as well, such as bathing a child, making the bed, and even applying your makeup. With a Web site like this at hand, you'll soon graduate summa cum laude in workout knowledge, at the top of your class and the bottom of your weight expectation.

The High Price of Firm

Now that you know just how many calories you burn off working out, you should know one more thing: It's gonna cost you! In an era of desk jobs and remote controls, exercise can be quite a pricey undertaking. Back in the Victorian era, people knew that you were a person of affluence if you had pale skin. Skin that was alabaster white meant that you had enough money to stay indoors instead of working outside of the home like a commoner. More recently, long fingernails were seen as a sign of wealth because it meant that you had enough money to pay someone else to clean your house, tend to your garden, and, I guess, pick your nose. Nowadays, a symbol of wealth is to have a muscular, cut body. This is due to the fact that except for those people who work in construction or dance in a cage, being in shape involves a health-club membership, a home gym, trendy bottled water—and, of course, enough narcissistic desire to spend all day working on yourself.

Now that we're in the twenty-first century, you show them the money every time you show them your ripped abs. Considering that the average price for a yearly gym membership is $250, the average price of a private trainer is $50 an hour, and the average price of a Juicy Couture tracksuit is $150, you can understand the high price of being firm. The way our economy is today, most Americans would have to choose between getting food or getting fit. Exercise doesn't have to involve a personal trainer and a liter of geothermal water, though. There are plenty of cost-cutting shortcuts that will allow you to beef up your muscles without atrophying your bank account.

1. Instead of buying a set of pricey exercise dumbbells, fill up your old plastic bottles with water and use them as weights.

2. Instead of hiring a personal trainer, buy a variety of workout tapes. Sure, you may not get the same level of workout, but you'll save an average of $150 a week for three hours of exercise, and that alone may motivate you to work out that much harder.

3. Instead of step classes, try climbing actual steps. Believe it or not, it burns just as many calories and works out the same muscles. Surprising, huh?

4. Instead of buying an expensive home treadmill, get an elliptical machine instead. They usually cost much less and can even be much quieter, so you're able to watch *Live with Regis and Kelly* without having to blast the volume.

5. If you want six-pack abs, put an actual six pack on your chest when you do your crunches. The added weight will make them much more effective. Not only is it a whole lot cheaper than buying an Ab Lounge or any other specially designed stomach-crunching machine, it's a lot tastier, too!

6. Finally, forget that expensive bottled health water from the Swiss Alps. Remember, fish poop in the water in Switzerland, too.

I'll admit it. I'm jealous of all those wealthy people who can afford a home gym and a personal trainer and have all that free time to focus so much energy on themselves. I read that Sarah Jessica Parker credits regaining her swimsuit-ready figure just months after giving birth to the fact that she could pay people to work her body and watch her kid. Few of us have that luxury. But, if we're creative enough and have enough motivation, we too can have a hard body, although we'll still have to take care of our own children, even when they're bratty. For that, I'll always be just a wee bit jealous.

Excuses, Excuses!

The high price of exercise is just one of the many excuses people can give for not working out. But the biggest excuse of them all is that people don't have enough time to exercise. Personally, I use that excuse more often than "Not tonight, dear, I have an irritated cornea" (my husband was getting sick of the headache excuse). When it comes to exercise, people complain that they're too tired to work out in the morning, too exhausted to work out at night, and too busy to work out during the day. My theory is that people find the time to do what they want to do, and if I told you I'd give you one million dollars to work out three times a week, you'd get your ass moving faster than Tommy Lee did in his infamous honeymoon video with Pamela Anderson.

The fact is that it does take time to work out. And I'm not just talking about the workout session itself. It takes time to mentally prepare yourself, time to get dressed (twice as long if you have to squeeze into anything made of spandex), and time to get to the exercise location site. Then you have to find a parking spot, drive home when you're done, and take that crucial postexercise shower. Often times, the whole process surrounding the workout can take longer than the workout itself.

On the flip side, I've never heard anyone complain that they're just too busy to watch TV. No matter how hectic someone's day turns out to be, they always seem to find the time to veg out on the sofa and watch endless hours of television. It may surprise you to know that the average person manages to squeeze in approximately four hours of television per day! Which of course proves my point: people do what they want to do.

Now don't worry, I'm not suggesting that anyone give up their sacred time with *Two and a Half Men* to do butt tucks. What I am suggesting is that you can incorporate exercise into your normal routine of television watching. If you take into account that the average half-hour prime-time show contains about ten minutes of commercials, you could work out for more than an hour a day if you'd just work out during each commercial break. You could do stomach crunches during one break and lunges during the next. In no time at all, you'd have a toned body and extra cash in your bank account because you hadn't watched all those advertisements that would have otherwise tempted you to buy products you don't really need . . . like those vacuum-sealed plastic bags that allow you to pack a whole winter wardrobe in one suitcase. (The problem being that when you pack for your return trip, you need to have a vacuum with you to get all the clothes to fit back in.)

By the way, according to my calculations, even after working out for that hour, you'd still have an extra twenty minutes of commercial time left to do other chores that you claim to be too busy to do, like dusting or washing the dishes. Ehh, who am I kidding? We're all too busy for that kind of stuff. Besides, some commercials can actually be quite entertaining, like the one about how things that happen in Vegas, stay in Vegas. That one always makes me giggle.

An Uphill Battle All the Way

There's nothing as wonderful as the feeling of being in really great shape. I was in really great shape once. It only lasted for a day, but oh, what a great day it was. I was in college and feeling sad and lonely and far away from home. I went to UC Santa Barbara and never really felt like I fit in. I didn't have blonde flowy hair and I couldn't hang ten on a surfboard. I couldn't even get tan since I was born with the kind of skin that only burned and then peeled (this is considered a hardship when you live in Southern California, and even allows you to park in the handicapped spots).

Then one day when I was walking along the beach feeling sorry for myself, I had a sudden and inexplicable desire to run to a far-off and distant pier. Of course, I was only able to run for a few minutes the first time I tried it, since I was hopelessly out of shape, but after weeks of daily effort, my body was finally strong enough to make it all the way to the pier without even getting winded. As I ran barefoot through the sand, I felt empowered, strong, and more alive than ever. And, as I finally touched my hand on that old weathered pier, I got an overwhelming sense of accomplishment (as well as some nasty blisters due to the hot sand on bare feet thing).

Unfortunately, that would be the last time I ever would touch that pier, because after that amazing day, I never ran back there again. I guess the wonderful feeling of being in shape wasn't enough to overcome my self-destructive need to abandon things once I finally attain them, which is why I always seem to gain back the weight after I struggle to lose it (but more about that later on). As the weeks went by, I felt my muscles shrink like a wool sweater in a hot dryer, and eventually, I couldn't even drive to the stupid pier without getting winded.

If you've ever been in great shape, then you know just how good it feels. But even though it's a great sensation, getting there is a near impossibility. That's because even though exercise is good for your body, your body seems to fight it every step of the way. You'll notice that when you first start working out, your body protests loud and clear. Your sides cramp and your lungs ache from not getting enough oxygen. Your muscles shut down and your whole body feels shaky. But if you're determined enough, you'll ignore these signs and keep on truckin', and after a while, you'll be able to see some progress. You notice that you can work out for a longer period of time without getting winded. You'll see that your once-loose muscles are getting tighter. Yes, after all your hard work and sweat, you'll feel like Rocky Balboa running up that legendary flight of stairs.

But then the challenges of staying in shape set in, as they always seem to do, which in turn makes you want to throw in your sweaty towel. For instance, perhaps something happens that makes you take a break from working out. Maybe you come down with a cold, or have to go on a business trip. Maybe you twist an ankle during a long run or your iPod needs repair. Whatever the reason, it's something that causes you to stop your routine for a certain block of time. And then when you're able to start up again, you find that your body's ability to work out has slipped back to where it was when you began. Yes, just by missing a few sessions, it feels as if you've never exercised at all, and trying to get back into shape becomes H-E-double-toothpicks. My theory is that deep down, my body really wants to be out of shape, and who am I to tell it otherwise?

Or, perhaps you work out regularly and do everything by the book, but it still takes forever for you to see any results in your appearance. After running enough miles to cross the country and doing enough lunges to catapult yourself into space, your muscles may lack that cut and defined look. Sure, you're able to work out longer without getting tired, but who the hell cares, if it doesn't make you look sexier in a tank top?

The reason that it's hard to see any results is that your muscles are covered by a layer of fat (in my case, it's more like a down comforter), and this layer needs to be shed before much definition can show through. That's why exercising when you're heavy is really a far less rewarding endeavor than doing so when you're thin. But as you know, it's important to combine both diet and exercise if you want your muscles to be as well cut as a Marquise diamond.

As you can see, getting in shape can really be an uphill battle all the way. But if you ever do stick it out and accomplish this miraculous feat, I hope that you can enjoy the incredible feeling of being in great shape for longer than just a day. And if you do ever run in the hot sand, make sure you wear shoes. Those blisters can be a real bitch.

Bally and Curves and Crunch . . . Oh My!

Now that you've educated yourself about working out and found the time to squeeze it into your day, it's time, as Nike says, to Just Do It. When it comes to getting a wide range of exercise choices, there is nothing that beats going to the gym. Because of the epidemic number of overweight people these days, there is also an epidemic number of gyms to choose from. Most all popular gyms today offer a wide variety of machines, weights, and classes to choose from for one low monthly fee (or at least that's what they say in their ads, but I've learned that they always have a little something hidden up their sleeves). Unfortunately, these gyms also offer a number of diverse problems.

To begin with, you can often spend more time trying to find a parking place than you spend working out. Then, when you do finally find a spot and go inside, you're overwhelmed by the stench of the place. Even with the ventilation system, it still smells as if you've walked into a warm armpit. You try not to faint as you make your way to your chosen piece of equipment, but inevitably, there's a line of people waiting to use it that's longer than that of any *Star Wars* premiere. When you finally do get your turn, you're only allotted a fraction of the time that you want to use it for. Not only is there a timer on the machine, but also a dozen people looking at you, making it impossible for you to work out long enough to see any results. Then, when you're through working out, you make your way into the locker room, which is more crowded than the King Tut exhibit. It's there that you're forced to get dressed in such close proximity to your neighbor that it's not uncommon for the two of you to inadvertently exchange some bodily fluids.

One common complaint of women who go to the gym is that they feel terribly self-conscious. They feel that all eyes are upon them during their workout. The men stare when they're in a compromising position on the inner thigh machine, and women stare at each other's trouble zones and mentally chant, *"There but for the grace of God go I."* Some, on the other hand, don't mind being ogled at the gym; in fact, they actually seek it out. They put on makeup and jewelry and seek out friends and colleagues. Me, I find the only person I ever run into is an old boyfriend who once broke my heart. I'm sure that after seeing me with my stringy hair, my bouncing fat, and that lovely stain of sweat just below my breasts, he's convinced more than ever that dumping me was the best decision he ever made.

But above and beyond any of those problems, the most offensive thing about the gym is the rude and gross behavior that fellow gym members exhibit. For some unexplained reason, they see the gym as their own personal haven and feel free to commit many offensive behaviors, such as these:

- People don't wipe off the machine when they're done, so you're greeted by a warm puddle of sweat when it's finally your turn.
- People talk loudly to their neighbors and you're forced to listen to their conversations about genital herpes or the ending of a movie that you were going to see that night.
- Men occasionally commit the inexcusable fashion error of wearing short shorts and no underwear.
- People sing along with their headphones in such a loud and abrasive manner that it makes even William Hung seem like an *American Idol*.
- Men have the tendency to grunt in a disturbing sexual nature when they work out hard.
- People don't always put the equipment back in the right place. If you're a neat freak, this can be quite unnerving.
- People come late to class and set up their mat right in front of you, blocking your coveted mirror space.
- People wear an overwhelming amount of perfume or cologne as if confusing the stomach crunch machine with a red-carpet moment.

The only way that going to the gym is ever a pleasant experience is if you're fortunate enough to be able to go during nonpeak hours. That way, you don't have to wait for the equipment, you don't have to get to classes early, and you don't have to risk contracting some kind of disease whenever you get dressed for the office. So if you're lucky enough to get fired or downsized, don't be depressed because you can no longer afford a roof over your head. Instead, think about how lucky you are that you can finally use the triceps machine for as long as you want.

Walk till You Drop

If the gym isn't your style, try going for a walk. In fact, walking is easily the most popular form of exercise of them all. It's easy to do, very low impact, and you don't need a trainer to teach you any complicated moves unless you've just awoken from a coma. There are amazing reported health benefits to walking, including lowering your risk of heart attack, cancer, and osteoporosis and increasing your good (HDL) cholesterol level. It's also cheap to do, since you don't have to buy any equipment or pay some extravagant membership fees (although there are some hidden fees, like the 800 iTunes downloads at 99 cents a pop).

Most of us already incorporate some amount of walking into our everyday life, which is a good thing because those experts who recommend things tell us that we should all do at least thirty minutes of moderate walking each day. If you add together the amount of time we walk from our car to our office, from our office to our lunch meeting, and from our driveway up to our front door, it should add up to a good four minutes' worth. Now we just need to find some way to incorporate that additional twenty-six.

When it comes to walking, there are two popular ways to go about it. The easiest method is to simply put on some overpriced sneakers, open up your front door, and take a nice long walk around your neighborhood. At first, you'll look forward to your daily treks down the sidewalk. Walking can be a very pleasant experience, and you'll be surprised at how many people, children, and dogs you'll meet along the way that you never knew lived in your community. Not only will walking make you feel like you're a part of your neighborhood, it just may score you some cool invitations to some hot summer BBQs.

But unfortunately, it won't take long before the mind-numbing boredom of walking sets in. Once you've counted how many squares there are on the sidewalk and mentally remodeled every home in your neighborhood, there's really not much left for you to do. Certainly, you can wave hello to your newfound friends, but that still leaves a lot of empty time to fill in between.

Soon, you'll be waking up in the morning and praying for rain so that you don't have to take your morning walk. Sure, you could make things more interesting by finding a neighbor to walk with. If she turns out to be a nice person, you'll find that the time will go by much faster due to your stimulating conversation. And if she turns out to be a loser, you'll find that you walk twice as fast to get home before she goes on about her recent hemorrhoid procedure.

If walking out in the real world doesn't appeal to you much, you can try the other popular method of walking: a treadmill. Although it is an effective method of exercise, it's far more expensive to buy a treadmill than a pair of tennies. Also, this method of exercise can be even more tedious than the first. On a treadmill, there's really nothing much to look at that would hold much interest, unless of course you set the thing up in front of Brad Pitt's rear end. At some point during your workout, you'll feel like a gerbil spinning around in its endless wheel. And the worst part of all is that when you exercise on a treadmill, you can't use the weather as an excuse not to work out each day.

Yes, walking may indeed have enormous health benefits, but it's still as dull as dirt to actually *do*. It may have been a big adventure when we were a year old and walked into our Daddy's waiting arms while everyone cheered. But somehow over the years, walking has lost a great deal of its allure, along with similar challenges like using a spoon and finding our thumb. But that doesn't mean that we don't have to do it. To keep ourselves fit, we still need to put one foot in front of the other, open that door, and take a walk. If we don't, we'll miss out on a lot of health benefits and a lot of great music downloads!

Yoga

Although no one is quite sure when yoga first began, some experts believe that it started as far back as 5,000 years ago. Although it's always been popular around the world, it was never very popular with me until I saw Madonna announce that yoga had become her exercise of choice on Oprah's show several years ago. Madonna and I are almost the same age, so I figure that if yoga can get her body in tiptop shape, it should be able to do the same for mine. Besides, how tough could it be to lie on a mat for an hour and stretch? As it turned out, it's as tough as cheap stew meat.

If you've never taken a yoga class, you can expect that your first class be quite a different experience than your usual exercise regime. In fact, in many ways, yoga is the complete opposite of the traditional experience you'll find at a modern-day gym. For instance, instead of smelling like an armpit, a yoga studio has a pungent smell of patchouli, or clover, or whatever other overpowering incense they decide to burn that day. And instead of loud, pounding music, they play only soft, instrumental New Age tunes. Even the language of yoga is unlike any you've heard at the gym before. The yoga instructor speaks in a different tongue than that used in a traditional workout environment. Instead of terms like "reps," "crunches," and "squats," you will hear things like "namaste," "ashtanga," and "chakra." The first time I listened to a yoga instructor, I was as lost as when I try to understand what the person is saying through the fast-food drive-through speaker.

The actual exercise of yoga is quite a bit different than the kind you get in a gym as well. Yoga is not about working your muscles to the point of exhaustion. It emphasizes stretching and lengthening and contorting your body into positions that can only be achieved by Gumby. But the biggest difference by far is that yoga emphasizes relaxation. In fact, that last fifteen minutes of yoga class is spent lying down on a mat while listening to relaxing music. Although it was rather calming, it was also rather disturbing, because many people were a bit too relaxed and farted freely throughout

❝ I feel like such a loser whenever I go to my yoga class. Everyone else is so limber and can bend their bodies in the most unnatural positions. I wasn't aware that you needed to have your spine removed before going to a yoga class. ❞

—Allison

the room. Oh . . . now I understand the whole burning incense thing.

There aren't any steel machines or heart-rate monitors in a yoga class either. Instead, there are soft bolsters and smooth blocks that allow you to stretch hidden muscles that you don't normally stretch a given day. And when you're not using the bolster or the block, the instructor makes you contort into positions that are illegal in several areas of the conservative South. By far my least favorite position is unfortunately the one that's the most popular. It's called downward dog, and to do it, you have to get down on your hands and feet and push your butt high in the air and as far back toward your feet as possibly. You look just like a dog when it stretches after taking a nap. I find this position quite uncomfortable for creatures who don't chase their tail or hump throw pillows.

The only time that I ever had fun during a yoga class was when my usual instructor was absent and the guy who played Michael Mancini on *Melrose Place* filled in for him. I guess "Michael" teaches yoga now as a way to fill in the time waiting for his *Melrose Place* residuals. I always had a crush on the guy, even though he married, divorced, and backstabbed every woman in that apartment complex, and he still looks pretty darn terrific today. During class, I found myself purposely getting into wrong positions just so he'd come over and correct me.

But except for those few memorable moments, I found that most of the yoga classes I attended lasted longer and were harder than I had expected them to be. Now I know why Madonna looks so good, and also why she looks so relaxed. Not only has yoga given her strong and lean muscles, but those relaxing last fifteen minutes of class no doubt relieved the pressure in her system from eating all that high-fiber Kabbalah food.

Must Not See TV

At first, the idea of having a workout instructor right on your own TV seems too good to be true. You don't have to worry if you lose your membership card. You don't have to wear cute matching outfits to class. And you don't have to carry around a bottle of trendy water so that people will think you care about your health when in truth, you just keep refilling the empty bottle with tap water. But as usual, if something seems too good to be true, it usually is, and home workout videos are no exception to the rule.

Workout videos have been around for as long as videotape machines. When I bought my first exercise video years back, Jane Fonda dominated the market. I was amazed at how convenient it was to work out at home and how nice it was not to have to schlep to the gym an hour before my aerobics lesson just to assure myself a spot in class. And best of all, I could do my butt lifts in front of the tube without having to deal with ugly men leering at me with Grinch-like looks on their faces.

Workout videos have come a long way, baby, since the early days of Jane Fonda. For one thing, they're now DVDs instead of videos. Also, the stores are filled with exercise options from Tae Bo to pole dancing. But no matter which exercise DVD you decide to take home with you, you can expect the same universal problems to occur with each and every one.

To begin with, you put the DVD in the machine, press the play button, and within a few warmup stretches (or hip gyrations if you decided upon a pole-dancing tape), you realize you forgot to get water. So you pause the machine and head to the kitchen to get a glass. You start up the machine again, get going on the floor routine, and the next thing you know, the telephone rings. You pause the machine again, answer the phone, and spend the next fifteen minutes trying to convince your boyfriend that, despite the fact that you're breathing hard, he didn't just catch you having sex with someone else. After you placate him, you hang up the phone, start up the tape, and get into the groove once more. But before long you hear the mailman at the door and know full well that he's putting this week's issue of *People* magazine in your mailbox. Within moments you're kickin' back on the sofa with a fresh bag of Cheetos, looking at a close-up of some actress's ass fat in full, glossy color while the video workout instructor continues to belt out orders in the background.

As you can see, it's quite easy to get distracted during an exercise class when your instructor is only two-dimensional. But there are other problems besides this bevy of interruptions. Some instructors tend to go quite fast, and it's hard for a beginner to keep up. Others may tell you to start with your right leg, but the instructor starts with his right leg, which looks like his left leg on the screen since he's facing you, making your workout as confusing as this last sentence. With other exercise videos, you fail to notice that you need to purchase additional equipment, like huge rubber bands or a giant exercise ball that makes you feel as small as an Oompa Loompa. Another big problem is that no matter which tape you buy, you'll soon have it memorized as well as *When Harry Met Sally*. When this happens, boredom is not far behind. Finally, when you're in an actual three-dimensional class, you're forced to do the whole routine. If you hate stomach work, you still have to plow through in a real class. But with a home exercise tape, you have the magical power of forwarding through time with your remote control.

As you can see, home videos are not always the solution to getting a convenient, all-over workout. Sure, they have many advantages over other forms of exercise, but it takes much more discipline and motivation to get a workout that's equal to that of a real-life class. Even with all that said, I do recommend them. They usually play great upbeat background music for you to listen to when you read about various celebrities' ass fat.

Other Ways to Get Physical

Although walking, private gyms, yoga classes, and home videotapes are some of today's most popular methods of exercising, there are still plenty of other methods that are worth mentioning. For one reason or another, these additional types of exercise have special, inherent challenges that can make them a bit less popular than the rest, but they are still every ounce as sucky and therefore just as deserving of getting their proper recognition. So, here they are:

Swimming
There's really no other exercise like swimming. It provides a great cardiovascular workout that incorporates every major muscle group. As you glide through the water, you feel as aerodynamic as a futuristic car. And when you've finished your workout, you step out of the pool feeling invigorated and refreshed, albeit a little bit wrinkled from all that

time in the water. But, unless you have regular access to a pool, swimming can be a very hard exercise to keep up.

Although swimming really is a wonderful sport, I do find that there are some problems associated with it, the main one being that I have trouble submerging myself in water that's any colder than my body temperature of 98.6 degrees. If it is, I go in toe by toe, slowing down even more at the most sensitive areas. And when I'm finally submerged, I have yet another problem with swimming: I don't find that it's such a great way to lose weight. It's as if Mother Nature wants to keep swimmers big and buoyant like giant walruses so that we can better withstand the icy cold water. But then again, maybe I don't lose weight because I'm not working out as hard as I think I am. It's difficult to get an accurate readout on how hard I'm exercising when I can't see how much I sweat.

Swimming in a chlorinated pool presents other problems as well. It can leave your hair green, your ends split, your skin dry, and your eyes bloodshot. So in the end, your swim can make you feel great, but you end up looking like crap.

And finally, unless you have a pool in your own back-yard, you're forced to swim at a community pool, where you're at risk of experiencing the most painful downside of swimming: a pool full of overweight men wearing Speedos. It's a sight that can hurt your eyes more than any amount of chlorine ever could!

Average cost to build an inground swimming pool: $25,000.
Average cost of snacks to feed your deadbeat neighbors who constantly show up at your door to go swimming: $500.

Pilates

Pilates was created by a man named Joseph Pilates who, in 1926, set up his first studio, close to the New York City Ballet. He created a unique series of movements that worked both mind and body and soon became the exercise of choice for both Martha Graham and George Balanchine. Me, I never took much notice of Pilates until I saw Melissa Rivers credit it for giving her a washboard stomach, just months after giving birth. I had my daughter not long before Melissa had her son, but my stomach was less like a washboard and more like a mushy load of wash. So I thought I'd get my tummy a crunchin' and give Pilates a shot.

Joseph Pilates perfected his exercise equipment during World War I by rigging the springs of a hospital bed. This may not come as a surprise to those who've seen modern-day Pilates equipment, since the machine does bear an odd resemblance to a turn-of-the-twentieth-century torture device. I know that when my instructor was using it on me, I was in so much pain, I would have confessed any secret that I had sworn to keep.

As it turned out, I really liked my Pilates class. Even though the exercises were hard, I got a total workout that incorporated both toning and stretching. Unfortunately, the equipment is unique, which makes the workout hard to mimic at home. Sure, they sell Pilates workout tapes and various contraptions that you can use at home, but I found that they weren't nearly as good as being in an actual Pilates studio.

The reason I didn't stick with my Pilates instructor has absolutely nothing to do with how good the class was. In fact, the only problem I have with taking a private Pilates class is the price of taking the class itself. Private Pilates classes can be very expensive, which is one of the reasons so many celebrities have no problem boasting that it's their exercise of choice. In fact, I calculate that Melissa Rivers could have bought herself a dozen washing machines for the price she paid for her one washboard stomach.

Average price of a private Pilates class: $50.
Average price of a washing machine: $650.

Spinning

If there was ever a time that I felt close to death, it was during the one and only spinning class I ever attended. My friend Jennifer persuaded me to join her by going *on and on* about how wonderful the class was and how there was no better way to burn more calories than by spinning. Jennifer said that if I went to the class, I'd feel great all day, and then sweetened the deal by offering to buy me coffee afterward. So I thought I'd be a good little adventurer, and a very big mooch, and give the class a try.

Suffice it to say, things did not go as well as I had hoped. For one thing, Jennifer failed to mention that I'd be forced to rent special spinning shoes that contained the residue of hundreds of sweaty feet that had gone before me. I have a phobia of communal shoes in general after suffering a certain bowling incident back in 1978, when I found something rather disturbing in my imitation leather shoes. I won't go into gory details, but suffice it to say that the person who put it there must have eaten corn that day.

After I put on the shoes and locked them into the bike pedals, the class began. It was at that moment that I instantly remembered something about bike riding that I had

> **❝**I took my place on one of the bikes at the front of the
>
> spinning class and there were a ton of people behind me. I
>
> found out afterwards that my leggings had a split in the crotch,
>
> and as I was leaning over my bike, my ass had been exposed to
>
> everyone to see behind me.**❞**
>
> —Melissa

somehow managed to forget: I hate it. I find bike riding to be an extremely uncomfortable sport, and that's when my tenders are nestled snuggly in a padded banana seat. In spin class, you're forced to sit on a hard projectile that feels like a cross between going on a bike ride and getting a Pap smear. These hard projectile seats aren't much of a problem for the hard-core spinners in the class, but that's because they spend most of the class standing up on their bikes. But for a peon like me, well, let's just say that I now understand the enormous correlation between the popularity of the spinning movement and today's epidemic fertility problem.

If you do decide to venture into a spinning class, heed this warning: The most important thing for you to do is locate the tension knob that's located in the front of your bike. By turning this knob, you'll be able to control the amount of effort you'll need to make the pedals move. I didn't know about this all-important knob. I was so busy fighting off my urge to vomit that I didn't even think to ask if the tension could be adjusted. Had I known, I might not have hated my experience as much as I did.

But in the end, I stuck out the class and didn't get off my bike for the entire time (although this was mostly due to the fact that I couldn't figure out how to unlock my damn shoes from the pedals). In the end, Jennifer turned out to be right. I did feel great for the rest of the day. But it wasn't because of the hard workout I got during class. I felt great because I had escaped death. Of course, I didn't tell this to Jennifer. Heck, I deserved a free nonfat venti latte after my ordeal.

So if you're the kind of person who loves hard-core exercise, wearing communal shoes, and getting a deep uterine massage, then spinning class is definitely the sport for you. Me, I'll stick to the kind of exercise that is kinder and gentler to my internal organs and doesn't cause my life to flash before my eyes.

Average price of spinning class: $15.
Average cost of shoe rental: $3.
Average price of Pap smear: $25 copay.

Jogging

Jogging is one of those sports that can really be quite rewarding—*if* you can find the strength and stamina to stick with it. After months of stick-to-it-iveness, you finally get to a point where you can run for a long period of time without getting tired. It's a very freeing feeling, not unlike a horse running through a field or O.J. racing down the 405 Freeway in his Bronco.

But jogging does have its downside. To begin with, it's one of the highest-impact sports around, and can be quite hard on your knees. And, if you are a woman with a big chest, it can be equally hard on your boobs. I have spent many a year looking for that perfect sports bra that can lock my breasts in place like a house bolted to its foundation. But alas, all the sports bras I've ever tried simply mash my chest into one giant breast loaf. Now that they've invented a vaccine for chickenpox, science should focus its attention on solving this physical ailment.

Once they master the sports bra, they need to move on to perfecting the other necessity for getting a good run: a mobile music system. Sure, there are the ever-so-popular Walkman and iPod, but I've found that there are no music devices around today that are totally devoid of problems. They have yet to invent a pair of earplugs that actually stay in your ears when you run. They have yet to invent a pair of batteries that don't run out during your favorite song. And they have yet to invent a radio station that plays more music than it does commercials. I did try something new recently and bought a Walkman that was able to pick up reception from television shows as well as music. I found it quite entertaining to listen to the *Today* show when I ran in the morning, and found that I'd get an extra great boost of energy whenever they interviewed a stud muffin like Orlando Bloom or David Beckham. I even raced home in record time to actually see them on TV.

So if you have strong knees, firm breasts, and a good audio device, you may actually enjoy the experience of running. Oh, and you also need to have a good pair of running shoes. I say "running" because if you go to any shoe store these days, you'll find shoes that are specifically designed for certain activities, including walking, hiking, and cross-training. Who knows? Maybe someday, there'll be a "taking in a movie" shoe that has a secret compartment for sneaking in your own candy and a sole that won't stick to the tacky floor. Or maybe a "help your friend move" sneaker that automatically gives your foot a cramp right before it's time to move the heavy appliances.

Average price of cool running shoes: $80.
Mandatory music system: $25–$300.
Used Ford Bronco: $6,500.

Home Exercise Equipment

Although most of us would love to have a home gym of our own, few of us are able to do so. For one thing, the machines are bulky and take up a lot of space in the house, and for another, sometimes they can cost more than the house itself. But even with these disadvantages, plenty of people go out and purchase at least one piece of home exercise equipment each year in hopes of trimming down their figure in the comfort and privacy of their own home.

I understand how someone can give in to the temptation of buying these machines. I too have seen the infomercials with the hard-bodied spokespeople who work up as much sweat on the equipment they're selling as I do when I struggle to open up a bag of potato chips. Like you, I'm tempted to pay $19.99 a month for a Bowflex, a treadmill, or an Ab Lounge, so that I too can have a rock-hard physique. But after a few minutes, enough time has passed for me to come to my senses, and to finally open up that damn bag of chips. Somehow, after that, I forget about the whole thing.

But if you have the spare funds, the spare room, and the spare tire around your middle, then go ahead and get yourself a home gym. I'm sure that you'll set it up, learn how to use it, and for a while, have a wonderful time working out. Just be prepared for the inevitable because, after the novelty wears off, the machine will take on its second life as it becomes a coat rack or dirty-laundry holder. In fact, that's what the commercials should really advertise these gadgets as. They should say, "A Bowflex has a unique lat bar that will not only strengthen your back, but is long enough to dry up to ten bras at the same time!"

If you're looking for a good way to save on home equipment, I suggest that you shop for it at garage sales or second-hand stores. I know there's something exciting about working out on a new, sparkling clean machine, but since I estimate the average time span from treadmill to coat rack to be 3.2 months, it makes good financial sense to buy cheap. Besides, while you're at these inexpensive places you can also pick up some embroidered tea towels and a few enchanting garden gnomes that you suddenly can't live without.

Average price of treadmill: $1,500.
Average price of actual coat rack: $100.

Alternate Uses for Home Exercise Equipment Once You Stop Using It

Before you go out and buy that big-ticket piece of workout equipment, you really should consider its afterlife and combine it with some of your other household needs. Here is a list of some of the double-duty activities home exercise equipment can provide:

- A treadmill is a great way to walk your dog when it's raining outside, or you're just too lazy to get off your ass and do it yourself.
- A yoga mat is good for laying out delicate sweaters to dry.
- Your larger-sized dumbbell makes an excellent panini sandwich. Simply make your favorite meat-and-cheese

sandwich, butter the outside of the bread, and put it on a hot griddle. Put a heatproof plate on top of the sandwich and weight it down with the dumbbell. Once the bread is brown and crispy, flip the sandwich over and cook the other side until the bread is cooked and the cheese is all melty and gooey.

- The timer on your stair climber makes a convenient spare kitchen timer whenever you're cooking several meals at once, like at parties or on Thanksgiving.
- An Ab Lounge makes a good, albeit not very sturdy, chaise lounge to go next to the pool. Use it for someone who comes to visit that you don't want to stay very long.

Feel the Burn(Out)

No matter which of the exercise plans you decide to choose, you'll find that you'll have one recurrent problem: boredom. True, whenever you first start a diet, you have a lot of motivation to work out. You choose your specific exercise plan and perform it religiously. You don your sweats and take a brisk walk around the neighborhood, or you put on your organic hemp pants and take a yoga class. But after a few short weeks, you find that you desperately want to quit. Yes, my friends, the exercise program that used to fill you with renewed invigoration now only fills you with complete and total boredom.

You try to get a quick boost, a motivation. You treat yourself to an expensive exercise top or some new CDs for your Discman, but the life span of this fix is shorter than the length of a micro-miniskirt. That's because no matter how much fun something is, it doesn't take long for it to become as dull as that part of the Oscars when those two accountant guys go over the voting rules.

Not only is doing one exercise over and over again dull, but it also primarily benefits only one part of your body. For instance, when you walk, run, or hike you're mainly working out the muscles in your lower body. When you use hand weights, it's only good for your arms, shoulders, and back (except of course if you're using them for doorstops, in which case they're only good for keeping a nice cross-breeze going).

There is a simple solution: Do more than one kind of exercise. (Duh!) Not only is this method much better for your mental health, but it's also much better for your physical health. When you alternate your workout routines, you won't have the same problem with boredom as you did before. You'll constantly be challenging new muscle groups and exposing yourself to additional stimulation, like the hunks at your new gym or the cutie-pies in your spinning class. Also, if you vary your workout, you'll no doubt have fewer injuries from repetitive motions and get better results overall, because cross-training works out your head, shoulders, knees and toes, knees and toes.

For some good options, try walking while carrying hand weights, riding your bike to your yoga class, or stopping to do some pushups at several points during a hike. Not only will you feel the burn, you'll feel much less burnout as well.

Send It Off in a Letter to Yourself

If you need a kick in the pants to get going, there's no one better suited to give it to you than you are. Believe me, no one wants to exercise. Well, maybe there are those few sado-masochists who actually enjoy torturing themselves with exercise and doing things like eating really hot peppers that make beads of sweat form on their foreheads. But as much as most people don't want to exercise, everybody loves having done it. They love feeling energized and healthy, and they love that radiant glow that can only come from exercising, being pregnant, or living next to a nuclear waste plant.

So why is it that getting yourself to do something that makes you feel wonderful is so incredibly difficult to do? It's not that way with other pleasures in life. Getting a relaxing massage requires no effort at all. And I don't see anyone ever complaining about getting a good old-fashioned mani-pedi. But getting yourself to work out requires at least a dozen reps of "I *really* don't want to do this!" and "I *really really* don't want to do this!"

If this sounds like you, I have an idea that just might help. I suggest that you write a letter to yourself as soon as you're done with your next workout. Get out a paper and pen and jot down how incredible you feel after your run or your step class or your hike. Write about how happy you are that you forced yourself to exercise. Don't forget to mention how your workout got rid of your blahs, and how strong and healthy you now feel, and how it really cured your craving for an Egg McMuffin.

When you're done with the letter, put it somewhere where you can read it before your next workout. For instance, if you go to a gym, keep it in your glove compartment so that you can read it while you're cursing in the parking lot about how much you really don't want to go inside. This little note that you wrote to yourself may just give you the additional motivation you need to get out of your car.

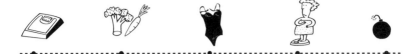

chapter six

motivational tools of the trade

A few years back, I heard a story on the news. It was a heart-breaking tale of a young girl who was dying of kidney failure. The only family member who was a compatible donor turned out to be her father. Unfortunately, he was morbidly obese, which meant that he was not a good candidate to be an organ donor because there was a chance that he wouldn't survive the operation. For decades before, the father had struggled with his weight, but could never find the motivation to lose it. Once he found out that he alone could save his daughter's life, he lost the weight as fast as Renee Zellweger did after she finished shooting *Bridget Jones's Diary*. He had the operation, pulled through beautifully, and today both daddy and daughter are alive and happy.

This story not only demonstrates a point, but it also adds a compelling tale to a book that's otherwise lacking in compelling tales. I'd bet that if faced with the decision to save a loved one or be the customer of the month at Burger World again, you too could manage to take off some weight. But for those of us who are not faced with such a conundrum, we have to find another way to get the motivation we need.

In general, people are motivated to diet for two distinct reasons—some by pleasure, others by pain. Some pleasurable reasons to start a diet would include being able to fit into a favorite outfit again, going to a vacation resort and not having to sit in a lounge chair the whole time, or going to a high school reunion being still worthy of your senior year title: "Girl Most Likely to Cause a Traffic Accident." Some painful reasons to diet would include the actual physical pain of sore knees and a sore back due to carrying around all that extra weight, or running into an acquaintance and being asked which trimester you're in.

But no matter what the reason is that made you go on a diet in the first place, I'm here to talk to you about motivation. We'll discuss various ways to get it, and more important, how to keep it. Just think of this chapter as a softcover Tony Robbins seminar without the ticket price, huge crowds, or souvenir T-shirts!

The Scales of Injustice

When it comes to a motivational tool, the scale can be a double-edged sword. If, after a few days of strict dieting, you step onto the scale and find that you're down a few pounds, you're as happy as a pig in . . . a warm cozy blanket (sorry, I can't use swear words if I want this book to sell at Wal-Mart). All of your hard work and your low fat intake has finally paid off. You raise your head high, and zip your pants higher, and are filled with enough motivation to last you through yet another week of dieting. To paraphrase James Brown, "You feel good!"

But if, after several days of dieting, you step onto the scale and it doesn't tell you what you want to hear, you sink into an abyss of depression that's lower than the price of Enron stock. For whatever reason, that vicious scale tells you that you didn't lose the amount of weight that you were hoping to lose. Or maybe you didn't lose any weight at all. Or worse still, maybe you actually put on a few pounds! When that happens, you're tempted to throw in the dieting towel and dive headfirst into a container of butter pecan. People who have been down the dieting road before know all too well that the scale can be a huge weapon of mass destruction for a diet. That's why many dieters go to one of two extremes when it comes to getting on the scale.

One extreme is to avoid the scale entirely during their diet. Instead of relying on a number on the scale to see if they've lost any weight, some people look for other signs, such as a looser waistband or fewer chins. They see if their ring can turn around on their finger, or if their belt is able to close on the second notch instead of the first. Personally, I agree with this theory but never have the inner strength to do it. I'm curious to a fault and would never survive a diet without getting on a scale (or a Christmas without opening up a few hidden presents).

Then there are people who exhibit the completely opposite behavior. Instead of avoiding the scale entirely, they insist on weighing themselves several times throughout each day. They weigh themselves when they first wake up in the morning, then again after breakfast, then before they leave for work, again when they get home, and finally, just before going to bed. They track their weight with the same diligence that men track baseball stats (sure, they can remember how many RBIs Randy Johnson had in a given season, yet they have no clue as to the date of your anniversary).

My cousin Meredith weighs in with the most frequency of anyone I know. She admits that she's obsessed with her weight when she diets, and it's not uncommon for her to get on the scale seven times a day. She feels that by doing this, she won't have any giant weight-gain surprises, and therefore feels more in control of her weight. I feel that she's being a bit obsessive-compulsive, but then again, I have that whole obsessive curiosity thing going, so I guess we're just one big mixed-up, wacky family.

So how often should you weigh in? Most experts agree that you shouldn't get on a scale more than once a week. I don't proclaim to be an expert on the issue of scale frequency, but I do consider myself qualified to offer creative ideas on what to do before you hop on the scale so that you will weigh less. Of course there are some basic tips, like weighing yourself naked so that your clothes don't influence the outcome, and weighing yourself when you first wake up so that your Rootin' Tootin' breakfast special doesn't influence the figure either. But, in addition to those ideas, there are a host of other things you can do to help tip the scale in your favor.

1. Blow your nose until you see particles of gray matter.
2. Pluck your eyebrows, shave your legs and pits, and wax your bikini line. If you're really hairy, this could add up to quite a substantial figure.
3. Exfoliate your skin to get rid of millions of dead skin cells. If you're looking for big results, do it with a cheese grater.

4. Cut your fingernails and toenails. If you're particularly nervous that your midnight snack may influence the results, remove your nail polish as well.
5. Go to the toilet and excrete everything that's excretable.
6. Get an army haircut.
7. Remove your makeup. If you emulate the look of Tammy Faye Bakker, this tip alone may help you reach your goal weight.

Finally, remember that your menstrual cycle is a huge influencing factor as to what the scale can say. If you know you're eating less than you usually do and still end up gaining a few pounds, you may want to look at the calendar to see when you're getting your period. I know that there are many women who put a big red circle on the date when they last got their period. I don't do this myself, but I'm sure my cousin Meredith draws seven of them.

Cheater, Cheater, Pumpkin Pie Eater

More often than not, my diets last as long as Britney Spears's first marriage. I start off the first morning full of motivation. I sit down with my piece of low-carb bread with a wee bit of sugar-free jam, and contentedly make it through my first meal. Then something goes wrong. When lunchtime rolls around, I'm no longer happy with my second diet meal of the day of torn lettuce with a splash of balsamic vinaigrette. My stomach depends on me for its usual fare of starch, gluten, more starch, and eventually more gluten, and it protests loud and clear. When I diet, my stomach becomes Fletcher

Christian, I become Captain Bligh, and this is mutiny on the body!

The way the diet manifests itself is to throw me a one-two-three punch of hunger pains, feelings of denial, and intense cravings. When I get sucker-punched in this manner, I have no recourse but to give in and cheat. After going on so many different diets over so many different years, I've come to the conclusion that all diets must be Teflon coated, because they're impossible to stick to.

As many of you dieters can attest, once you take a mouthful of something fattening, you can kiss your diet goodbye. When your long-deprived tongue tastes something creamy, gooey, or crunchy, there's no turning back. It's like an ex-smoker having just one cigarette, or a sex-aholic having just one afternoon delight.

Everyone has their own scenario for when they're the most vulnerable to this one-two-three attack. With me, it's almost always a combination of several of the following factors:

- I've eaten less than I should have at one meal and am therefore fiercely hungry come the next.
- It's some time after lunch, yet before dinner . . . the danger zone of my day.
- I'm alone and therefore don't have to eat like a normal civilized person who wouldn't dream of eating a pudding cup with only her tongue.
- I'm dangerously close to a whopper of a temptation like homemade cookies, warm doughnuts, or an actual Whopper at my friendly neighborhood Burger King.

I can be strong if I have only one factor working against me, but when you stack all three together, I'm in deep doo-doo. At first, I reach for something healthy like an apple or a scoop of cottage cheese in an attempt to kill the craving, but that's about as helpful as taking a baby aspirin during hard labor. So I take a piece of the forbidden fruit (or in this case, fruit pie) and find it incredibly satisfying. It's like drinking water when you're really thirsty or peeing when you've held it in so long, your bladder is minutes away from infection. I try to stop myself but I can't. As fast as I can say "BHT as a preservative," I'm sitting on the sofa, watching bad TV, and using my finger to scrape out the last bit of imitation BBQ flavor from the bottom of my potato chip bag. I try to stop myself but there's no turning back. I invade my pantry like a locust on corn, devouring everything in sight.

As you know from experience, this is the danger point of any diet, and the time that having a strong motivation to lose weight is the most critical. Not long after you've had the last of the lemon meringue pie, the feeling of self-loathing takes over and you find that you're at a sugarcoated fork in the dieting road. Do you climb back up on the fat-free bandwagon or stay on the floor licking up all the fallen crumbs?

The diet experts would say that you should get right back on track. You had a setback and you need to forgive yourself. I myself have a hard time listening to experts, which is why I never rinse and repeat. But I do believe that they're right about this one. I too believe that if you cheat, you should get right back on the diet. Granted, that's much easier said than done. You look down at your belly, which has plumped up like a warm Ball Park frank. Soon, your sugar level will plummet, causing severe hunger pains, and you'll be filled up with more gas than an oil refinery. Most of all, you'll be tempted to cheat again and blow your diet for good.

This is the circle of life, my friend—a dieter's life, that is. And this circle has been spinning its wheel ever since the invention of marshmallow cream. But if you can find enough motivation, you should pick yourself up by the bootstraps on your bloated feet and keep on dieting. *Focus* on how far you've come. *Realize* that there'll always be setbacks in life. *Expect* that you'll cheat from time to time, so you won't be so distraught when it actually happens. What you need now is strong motivation, plenty of self-forgiveness, and maybe a bottle of Maalox for the gas.

Mix It Up

For many of us, falling into a rut is an easy thing to do. We watch the same TV shows week after week. We buy the same color car every few years. And we eat at the same restaurant every time we're lucky enough to find a good sitter. Yes, it seems that we've all become "vanilla" in a world of thirty-one flavors. That's why it comes as no surprise that when we diet, we fall into a consistent rut as well. We make ourselves the same low-fat breakfast of wheat toast and fruit (unless we're on Atkins, in which case it's a ham and cheese omelet). For lunch it's a green salad with low-cal dressing (unless we're on Atkins, in which case it's a double-cheese bacon burger). And for dinner it's the usual fare of a skinless breast of chicken with a side of steamed vegetables (unless we're on Atkins, in which case we're skipping dinner to have a triple bypass). The problem with this pattern is that people aren't built like dogs that can eat a steady diet of Alpo every day. We need variety in our lives to keep things interesting, and if we don't have it, we become easily bored, and therefore, easily cheat.

It really doesn't matter what type of diet that you decide to go on. At first glance, the high-protein diets sound so wonderful. You could never imagine that you'd tire of bacon. But human beings can tire of anything that they have on a regular basis, no matter how wonderful it is, which explains why Rebecca Romijn was able to leave John Stamos. But the truth is that a person can only eat so many Cobb salads, protein-style burgers, and jerky sticks without getting bored.

Just as in our sex life, it's important to have some variety in our diet to keep things interesting. We need to seek out things to amuse us, whether it be edible flowers or edible panties. When it comes to your diet, keeping things interesting will motivate you to stick to your diet longer. Instead of eating the same boring entrées day in and day out, make each meal a brand new adventure. It's important to spice things up, even if it's as simple as putting different spices on your food. Here are some simple adventures you can try:

- Instead of your usual dull turkey sandwich, wrap the turkey into a whole-wheat tortilla, sprinkle on some low-fat cheese, heat it up in the microwave and, ¡ole! You have a tasty burrito.
- Instead of boring steamed vegetables, put them in a blender with some nonfat milk and herbs and make a creamy soup.
- Instead of plain fruit from the refrigerator, heat things up a bit. Take a plain peach, slice it in half and put it

on a hot grill. Or cut up an apple, sprinkle it with a dash of cinnamon, and bake it until it's as soft as pie filling. Same amount of calories, far more delicious.

- Instead of denying yourself dessert, have a fat-free or sugar-free Fudgsicle (depending on your diet of choice). If you want to cut calories even more, try a sugar-free Popsicle. These are only 15 calories each and really satisfy a sweet tooth!

- Instead of ice cream, try frozen grapes. Frozen blueberries are also great just poured into a bowl. If your diet allows, slice some bananas, wrap them in plastic wrap, and put them in the freezer. For an added zing, sprinkle a little cocoa powder on them before you freeze them so they'll taste like chocolate-covered bananas!

If you can find a way to keep things interesting, you'll find that you'll be able to avoid boredom and stick to your diet for a much longer period of time. And, if you can ever find those edible panties, you'll avoid boredom as well and find you'll be able to stick with your bed partner for a longer period of time too!

Diet Buddy

If it's true that misery does indeed love company, then a diet is an excellent time to take a friend along with you. These "diet buddies" can be a wonderful tool to keep your motivation level high. When you have a diet buddy, you can take hikes together and compare recipes. You can call each other when a strong craving hits and go to holiday parties together to slap each other's hands if they reach for one too many Cheez Doodles. Yes, a diet buddy can be a wonderfully supportive asset to motivate you along on your diet. But she can also be a hindrance.

I had a diet buddy once but it didn't turn out to be the positive experience I had hoped it would be. For one thing, my diet buddy would never call me. I was always the needy one in our relationship. There were even times when I'd call her several times in one evening, usually the days when I'd catch up on *The Sopranos* (they always seem to be eating yummy things on that show). My diet buddy wasn't the most considerate diet buddy either, since she'd often forget to turn on her cell phone and therefore wasn't there for me when I would pass by the sample tray at Mrs. Fields. But the real atrocity she committed was that she was far more successful on her diet than I was, and would often lose twice the weight that I did each week. Within a month, my diet buddy got sick of my neediness and finally dumped me. We tried to remain friends, but it was too painful for me to see her in her size-four jeans.

> ❝I had a diet buddy who was way too demanding for my taste. She'd call me first thing in the morning and make me give her a list of exactly what I was planning to eat for the day. And if I ever strayed from that list, I had to call her immediately so that she could reevaluate things. It was like having Joseph Stalin for a diet buddy.❞
>
> —Amy

So take a lesson from me. Don't think that you can choose any full-figured person to be your diet buddy. First, when choosing a diet buddy it's important to select one who's heavier than you are. The last thing you want is someone to scale down faster than you do. Next, select a responsible diet buddy who has a well-charged cell-phone battery and ample minutes on her calling plan. And finally, just as with any partnership, you have to select a worthy opponent. For instance, when you're looking for a tennis partner, you want to choose someone who plays just a wee better than you do. This way you'll be challenged and can pick up some tips. The only thing you'll be picking up if you play with a lesser opponent is a multitude of unreturned tennis balls. My advice? Choose a buddy who's also a coworker. She's around you all day and you can support each other through tedious lunch hours filled with plain yogurt and celery sticks.

If you're looking for a diet buddy but can't seem to find one, or can't find one who's compatible, get an online pal. You can probably find a service that's free. The obvious problem with an online diet buddy is that it's a bit difficult for your cyberpal to take that double-dip cone out of your hands, but then again, you don't have to see her flaunting her new size-four jeans in front of you either.

The Write Way to Get Motivated

"Journaling" is a verb that's quite popular among those in the diet world. In case you're not fluent in the language of diet, journaling is the act of writing down everything that you consume throughout the day. And I do mean everything.

Every morsel of food that passes through your lips must be written down and accounted for in full detail, as if you were logging in the evidence of a crime scene. The reason that journaling can provide motivation for your diet is that it gives you a reference guide to reflect upon whenever you need incentive to keep on going. With your journal in hand, you have tangible proof that your body can indeed survive on 1,200 calories a day, you can consume five servings of fruits and vegetables in one twenty-four-hour period, and yes, it is humanly possible to go to The Olive Garden and not order the fettuccine Alfredo.

Although some diets, such as Weight Watchers, require journaling, it can be very beneficial for other diet plans as well. When you're forced to write down everything you eat, you suddenly become aware of all the cheating you do throughout a given day that you didn't even know you were doing. There were those potato chips that you munched on when you were packing your son's lunch, and those croutons from your Caesar salad that you just didn't have the heart to pick off. When I started journaling, I stopped blaming my slow metabolism for my weight gain and started blaming the sample bags of slow-roasted peanuts that I had at the bottom of my purse.

There are some people who are a bit more obsessed with journaling than the average dieter and who take it to a whole new level. In addition to filling in their food intake column, they also fill in a column that tracks their daily exercise. Every time they run for the bus or climb a flight of stairs, they make a note of it. At the end of the day, they add up the number of calories they consumed, subtract the calories they burned off with exercise, and hope they come out in the black.

My only advice when it comes to journaling is to not get too far behind. Ideally, you should head to your journal immediately after you finish your meal. I know I have a hard time remembering what I did this past weekend, let alone how many slices of fat-free ham I put in my sandwich for lunch two days ago. Two-thirds of my brain cells are already full of useless information like the words to the Peter Piper rhyme and the names of all my elementary school teachers. I have to keep the other remaining cells free for important information—things like how much bulk toilet paper I have left in the garage—so I find that I have to jot down my food intake as soon as I swallow or else the information is lost forever.

As you can see, journaling is a great way to add motivation to your diet, as well as a good source to turn to when you're trying to figure out why you're not losing the weight you hoped to lose. And if you suffer from the same lack of brain cells as I do, try aromatherapy. Or is it electrotherapy? I can never remember which one is which, which may explain why taking a lavender-scented bath is so painful.

As long as you're at it and journaling away, why don't you keep track of other details in your life that may help you down the line, such as these:

Keep track of how much money you saved by clipping coupons so that you can rationalize buying some ridiculously overpriced pair of shoes.

Keep track of how many minutes you spent talking to your mother-in-law so that when your mother wants to visit, your spouse has no right to complain.

Keep track of the gross things you do for your husband (popping the zits on his back, wiping off his pee that missed the bowl) so that when he gives you an attitude about clearing away the dinner dishes, you have ammunition for the big fight that will ensue.

Good Things Come to Those Who Weight-Loss

I'm not one who's big on patience. I'm into things like instant oatmeal and Minute rice. I go to one-day cleaners and 3 Day Blinds and detest all things that require me to stand in line for a long period of time. So as you can imagine, I have quite a difficult time waiting around to see the results of a diet. I know myself well enough to know that if I don't lose twenty pounds in one week, I'll feel like the diet isn't working, and I'll be tempted to quit.

I know what the experts would say. They'd tell me that I didn't put the weight on in one day, and that it's not going to come off in one day either. And even though I agree with their logic, that doesn't mean that I have to be very happy about it. To add insult to injury, these experts also advise that I shouldn't lose more than 2 pounds a week. Two pounds a week my ass. That's nothing. If I followed their advice, it'd take me a month just to lose the extra weight *on* my ass.

But those so-called experts believe that slow and steady really does win the weight-loss race. They think that if you lose anything more than 2 pounds a week, you're not just losing fat, but muscle as well. They also say that if you lose weight quickly, you're more likely to gain it all back, and then some, in the same speedy manner. Don't you just hate those experts? They sure suck all the fun out of diets, as well as other things, like basking in the sun all day.

Because you're really supposed to lose weight gradually, it's important to keep your motivation level strong throughout your diet. But that's something that's much easier said than done. How does one keep motivated for weeks or even months at a time? For me, there are only a few motivational factors that keep me on my diet track. One is when the scale tells me that I'm losing weight. Another is when my clothes get baggy. And the last is when I get a compliment on how good I look from people I know. As you can imagine, there's a whole lot of empty time in between that needs to be filled with a strong dose of motivation, especially when I'm in line at the checkout counter within an arm's reach of a Kit Kat bar.

If you're anything like me, you need a strong dose of motivation just to get out of bed in the morning, let alone stick to a diet. So let's get right down to it, shall we? Here are some invaluable tips on how to stick to your diet through the thick, and eventually, the thin:

1. Make yourself an "ugly" photo book. Gather up all those photos of yourself that you hate because you look fat in them, and combine them all into one book. Keep this book close by at all times for instant motivation.

2. Go to *www.Oprah.com* and order archive tapes of some past shows that deal with weight loss success stories. Type in "weight loss" in the Search box, and you'll

read all about dozens of past shows that you can order to inspire you.

3. Before you start your diet, write a note to yourself about what motivated you to go on the diet in the first place, and how being overweight makes you feel. Whenever you question whether all this work is really worth it, read the note. While you're at it, jot down how bad you felt after you cheated on your diet and read it the next time you're tempted to cheat again.

4. Take a digital photograph of your biggest trouble zone and use it as your computer screen saver. This will stop you from reaching into your snack drawer during office breaks.

5. Keep a powerful article of clothing out to view each morning when you're getting dressed. This could be the fat pants that you're so disgusted with, or it could be a dress that you long to fit into again.

6. Give yourself a regular stream of rewards. Buy yourself a gift either after losing a certain number of pounds or sticking to your diet for a certain length of time. The treats should be ones that make you feel good about yourself, like new makeup, a flattering sexy blouse, or professional highlights. Or, what the hell, make it a stunning diamond necklace with matching earrings. After all, dieting is hard!

7. Watch TV shows that show diet success stories, such as *Weighing In* on the Food Network, *The Biggest Loser* on NBC, or *Extreme Makeover* on ABC.

8. Give a nominal fee to your friends and family and ask them to keep those compliments a comin'! They really do make you feel terrific.

The most important thing about weight loss, as well as the most difficult, is to be realistic about just how long it will actually take for you to reach your goal weight. Personally, I think it's best to err in excess. Figure out how much you want to lose, calculate an average of only one pound a week just to be safe (and to average in a few unstoppable cravings for iced blended mochas), and see where that date falls. If you want to lose ten pounds, count on ten weeks to do it. By overestimating how much time it will take for you to reach your goal weight, you'll be setting yourself up for success. You don't have unrealistic expectations about losing it all in a couple of weeks. And you won't feel the need to quit if your computer crashed before you backed up your work and you numbed your pain with a sheet cake. If you ever do cheat, catching up is certainly doable, and best of all, the "one pound per week" makes calculations so darn easy! I know that it seems you'll need even more patience if you err on the side of excess, but then when you lose the weight ahead of schedule, you'll feel like the winner that you truly are!

Dream a Little Dream of a Littler You

If you think about it, dreams are miraculous events. Where else but in dreams can you write your own stories, design your own wardrobe, direct all the shots, build all the sets, and of course, be the star! And like all other Hollywood stars, you too can have the thin, emaciated, anorexic look that all actresses aspire to. All this makes dreaming a great motivational tool in a diet because dreams can enable you to see what you'll look like without the need for laxatives, enemas, high colonics, or any other Hollywood weight-loss secret.

When you're in la-la land, you can be anything that you want to be. If you're blind, you can see. If you're poor, you can be rich. And if you're heavy, you can be thin. In my youth, I used to love to have the dreams where I could fly. Now that I'm older, I love having the dreams where I'm slender enough to wear horizontal stripes. I can walk into any room and turn heads, and not because my wide ass just knocked something over. Whenever I have a fantasy dream like this, I awake full of excitement and motivation to attain my inner thin self so I can look as fantastic as I did in my dream.

The other kind of dream I look forward to having is the kind where I can eat myself into oblivion and not get full, gain an ounce, or feel the least bit guilty. Often, when I'm on a diet and go to bed hungry, I dream of stuffing my face full of fattening treats. I've satisfied my long-denied sweet tooth with mouthfuls of candy and platefuls of pie. I've had Double Stuf Oreo cookies and double-dipped cones. And like all my other dreams, it seemed so real that I felt like I got all the satisfaction, without any of the painful gas and bloating!

The only downfall to this wonderful state of euphoria is when you're awakened in the middle of one of these delectable dreams. If you were ever upset when you were awakened during a sex dream, just wait till you see how angry you'll be when you're awakened during a Tex-Mex dream in which you're stuffing your trap full of shrimp tacos and watermelon margaritas. Heaven help your kid if he wakes you up in the middle of that feast just because he saw a monster in his room. Oh, you'll show him a monster, all right!

The Most Wonderfully Fattening Time of the Year

You may have heard the expression the "Holiday 7," which is based on the long-standing urban legend that the average person gains approximately 7 pounds during the weeks from Thanksgiving to New Year's. Me, I've always considered myself a little above average, which is why I tend to gain at least 10. I don't know if the Holiday 7 story is true or not, and researching that fact would most likely cut into my TiVo time, but I do know that there are many things one can do to scale down this number.

To begin with, timing in life is everything. If you can, you should avoid starting a diet during these last two delicious months of the year. Planning a new diet around the holidays would be like planning your honeymoon around the start of your period. But if you must begin a diet during the holidays, be warned that you're going to need a heck of a lot of motivation to see you through till New Year's Day. So before you venture out to parties that involve Secret Santas and mistletoe, here are some extra-strength motivational holiday tips:

- Before you leave for any party, make sure that you eat a small healthy meal. This way, your stomach won't be so hungry and your hands won't be so tempted to grab some Jordan almonds while your drunken boss grabs your ass.
- Drink plenty of water throughout the event. If you can, pour it into a beautiful party glass and throw in a slice of lemon.
- Although my grandma would never agree with this one, chew a piece of gum while you're at the party.

As you can imagine, it's quite difficult to put a crab puff in your mouth when there's already a big wad of Carefree in there.

- If you must drink alcohol at the party, have a wine spritzer. That way, you get all the taste of wine with only half the calories.

- BYOD: I know this one may be awkward, but bring your own dressing. Dips and dressings are the death of many a diet and often contain as many fat grams and calories as dessert. You can easily find several different brands of low-cal dressings at the store that come in individual serving-size packets. Throw a bunch in your purse and use them in place of other dips, sauces, and of course, salads.

- As you know, holidays are a time of giving. So if someone gives you a tin full of frosted cookies or spicy cakes, pass it along to your neighbors or put it directly into the trunk of your car and take it to work the next morning. Yes, not only is it better to give than to receive, it's also a heck of a lot less fattening.

Bistro Binging

Another time when you need a little extra motivation to stick to your diet is when you go out to eat. I know how reluctant you can be to leave the safe, fiber-filled confines of your house and venture out into the real world, where extra-virgin olive oil flows so freely. At home you're restricted to the boring low-fat foods that occupy your fridge, but at a restaurant, there's a long list of temptations to choose from. It's like Club Med for your taste buds, but instead of being tempted by salsa music and blue, clean oceans, you're tempted by tomato salsa and blue corn chips.

I myself have blown many a diet by going out for dinner. Once the waiter sets down that basket of warm bread in front of me, I'm doomed. I try to keep it together, but I fall apart when I watch the bevy of delectable dishes being brought out of the kitchen. I feel like I'm a judge at a Miss Universe contest gawking at the array of mouthwatering selections strolling past me, like Maine lobster, New York steak, and Maryland crab cakes. Be still my heart!

I take a cleansing breath, browse the menu, and search for an item that fits into my diet plan. I salivate at the deep-fried appetizers and the cream-sauce temptations but stay strong and order the boring whitefish. Unfortunately, when it arrives, it's floating in a sea of melted butter. I pick out a bite and sop up the grease with my napkin, hoping to spare myself the extra million calories. But in the end my fingers are greasy, my stomach is hungry, and I'm pissed off that I just paid $17 for five bites of food. So I leave the restaurant and drive through the closest Taco Bell for a Gordita Supreme and vow not to leave my house until I've reached my ultimate goal weight, or until they make a low-cal version of that Gordita thing, because it really is to die for!

Unless you want to become an agoraphobic and have an anxiety attack every time you venture out into the real world to eat, you have to learn how to go to a restaurant and stay on track. Maybe some of these diet suggestions will help you down that path.

1. Go to a restaurant that is diet friendly. For example, Applebee's offers meals approved by Weight Watchers,

"Whenever I go out to dinner, my boyfriend calls me 'Sally' from that movie, "When Harry Met Sally", because I always order my dressing and sauces on the side. He says he's just being cute, but deep down I know it embarrasses him because he thinks I'm bothering the waiter. If you ask me, the real reason he calls me Sally is to stop himself from calling me a meaner name that would lead to a fight."

—Miranda

and Chili's has Guiltess Grill food selections that make the process easy.

2. Dress in something with a tight waistband. You'll be less likely to overeat when you know it would lead to cutting off the circulation to your legs.

3. Don't be afraid to ask questions. It's always a good idea to find out exactly how your meal is prepared and what it comes with. A lot of fancy restaurants use foreign names for food that may sound fattening when in actuality they just mean lettuce or squash.

4. To keep the portion size under control, order an appetizer-size portion instead of a full one, or look for items that allow you to get only a half order of that selection. Or better yet, just lap up the crumbs that are dropped on the tablecloth by your fellow diners.

5. Don't be fooled into thinking that just because you order a salad, your meal is going to be slimming. Be wary of hidden calories in creamy dressings, high-fat cheese, and croutons. A good tip is to get the dressing on the side, dip your fork into it, shake off the excess, and then stick the fork in the salad. This way you'll

have the taste of the dressing without a soufflé's worth of calories in every bite.

6. Don't be embarrassed to ask for a certain item on the menu to be cooked in a diet-friendly manner. Tell the waiter that you want your fish steamed instead of sautéed, or that you'd like your vegetables prepared with no oil. He doesn't mind a bit (or at least he has to pretend that he doesn't mind if he wants a nice tip).

7. Have a piece of fruit or a slice of fat-free cheese before you leave for the restaurant so that you won't be so hungry. I know it sounds odd to eat before you go out to dinner, but you clean up before the housekeeper comes and you don't think twice about that.

Weight-Loss Plateaus

There is evil all around us. Every freeway has a driver with road rage. Every high school has its dangerous gang. Every department store has a salesgirl who wants to douse you with stinky-ass perfume. But even worse than all of these monstrosities combined is the fact that every diet has a weight loss plateau that's waiting for you just around the bend. Any dieter who's ever gone the distance knows exactly what a weight-loss plateau is, but for those millions of other people whose diets last as long as a Macy's One-Day Sale, let me explain.

A weight-loss plateau occurs when your body loses a certain amount of weight and then, despite your best efforts and intentions, refuses to lose any more. At the beginning of most diets, the weight has a tendency to fall off of you like the meat from an overcooked pork rib. At this early stage, you're chock-full of motivation, as well as excess water weight. But several days and several pounds later, your body gets wise to the fact that you're trying to get rid of it—or at least part of it. You religiously adhere to every step of your diet but the scale refuses to budge.

What you have to understand is that from a survival standpoint, your body wants to stay overweight so that it can continue to live for a long period of time should your food supply run out (it obviously doesn't realize there's a Starbucks on every corner). When you diet, your body sees you as the enemy who's out to destroy it and holds on to its fat as tightly as a fishmonger holds on to stink. This, my friend, is when the weight loss plateau occurs.

A weight-loss plateau can be the death of any diet, especially if you're not motivated to get past it. But in addition to pure motivation, you also need some education. For one thing, you need to know that you can't possibly continue to lose the large amount of weight that you did at the beginning of your diet. One reason for this is that as you thin down, your body naturally needs less food to maintain itself. As you can imagine, a body uses fewer calories to sustain a thinner frame than one that's larger. For another, the smaller you are, the harder it is for you to drop as many pounds as you did when you were heavier. If a 200-pound person lost 10 percent of his body weight, that would add up to 20 pounds. But for a 100-pound person, it would be only 10. Also, you need to understand that if you're going to diet, a weight-loss plateau is as inevitable as having a big zit just in time for a hot date. If you expect it to happen, you won't be so upset when it occurs. Knowing these facts going into a diet just may make it easier to get through.

Believe me, if you have the strength to get past a weight-loss plateau, you have the strength to get past anything, for what doesn't kill you makes you stronger—and often, a whole lot thinner too. In fact, once you're past the plateau, you're prepared for any of these events:

1. A home remodeling in which everything that could possibly go wrong, does.
2. Having visitors who don't know about the "house-guests and fish go bad after three days" rule.
3. Plucking out those sensitive hairs on your toe knuckle.
4. Having the cable go out during Oprah's annual "Favorite Things" show.

Is There Such a Thing as Too Much Motivation?

Whenever any of us does something new, we have a tendency to get very excited about it. For instance, when I got pregnant, I read every book on the subject there was to read. I knew the day my baby developed her arms and legs, when she was able to hear things outside the womb, and when she took her first pee in the amniotic fluid. I was obsessed with doing everything right, which is why I abstained from drinking, smoking, drugs, and to my husband's despair, sex. Sure, the books told me that sex was okay, but I didn't want to take a chance of creating dimples where dimples don't naturally occur.

The same theory holds true for dieting. Often, when we start a new diet, we have these same feelings of excitement. We read our diet book from cover to cover, we cook healthy meals

> **❝**I knew I was getting too obsessed with my diet when I didn't want to lick the envelopes when I paid my bills. For all I know, they make that glue out of frosting!**❞**
>
> —Taylor

without adding even a smallest hint of added fat, and we learn to calculate calories and carbs as adeptly as Dustin Hoffman's character counted fallen toothpicks in *Rain Man*. But life is too short and dieting is too hard to live life this way.

Don't get me wrong. You should know what you're eating when you're on a diet. For instance, did you know that a healthy glass of orange juice has about the same number of calories as two cookies, and that a good-sized bite of a dense, creamy cheesecake can have as many as 100 calories? But if you've stopped biting your fingernails because you can't find the carbohydrate count of "nail" in any of your diet books, then you too may be a bit too obsessed with your food intake.

One obvious sign that you're too obsessed is that your friends stop taking your calls, just as they did when you got a new boyfriend and you made them listen to the cute messages he left on your machine over and over again. But other clues may not be as obvious. If you exhibit any of these behaviors, you may want to pursue other interests in your life besides your daily food intake to keep you occupied:

1. You abstain from taking over-the-counter medicine like Motrin simply because the bottle doesn't list the calorie count of a gel cap. Is it worth making your

jeans permanently tight just to get rid of some pre-menstrual cramps?

2. No matter how stinky your breath is when you diet, you pass when your coworker offers you a Listerine breath strip. Sure they're minty, but do those paper-thin wafers contain as many carbohydrates as a biscuit? The world may never know.

3. You know you don't eat a well-rounded diet, but you refuse to take a multivitamin. You'd hate to have the willpower to pass on dessert only to end up gaining weight anyway because of a little riboflavin and B12.

4. You're sexually active but refuse to take your daily birth control pill because you don't know how many calories it contains. What's a little unplanned pregnancy compared to some unplanned weight gain?

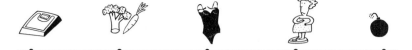

chapter seven

the blame game

Don't you just love it when you have a valid reason excusing you from doing something you really don't want to do? Like when you're excused from bringing anything to the office potluck lunch because your oven's on the fritz? Or when you're excused from serving jury duty because you're a stay-at-home mom and can't leave your young children alone no matter how much you're tempted to do so from time to time? And the best one of them all: when you're excused from being overweight because of some factor that's totally out of your control.

Look at Jerry Lewis, who blew up like an inflatable raft when he had to take steroids for his lung condition. Instead of judgments and looks and tabloid covers, all this deserving man got was sympathy and cards from well-wishers. But for those of us who aren't lucky enough to have an obvious medical condition to blame for our added weight, here are some possible no-fault-of-our-own excuses that we can use.

Metabolism Schmatabolism

In case you aren't aware of what a metabolism is, it is the rate at which a body breaks down food into energy. It's sort of like the efficiency of a car engine. For instance, if you drive a Hummer, it will take a lot of fuel for you to drive from point A to point B. But if you have a fuel-efficient hybrid, it won't take nearly as much fuel to travel the same distance. Two cars, one distance to travel, and two different amounts of fuel needed to get there.

Having a slow, Hummer-like metabolism is one well-recognized physiological reason for being overweight. Blaming a slow metabolism for those extra pounds is as socially acceptable as excusing an irate woman because she has PMS, or freeing a celebrity felon because he has enough money to hire a top attorney. It's a well-known fact that the rate of our metabolism directly affects what we weigh. We all know people who can eat whatever they want without getting fat—although we've permanently removed their numbers from our phone books. And we all know others who can move up three dress sizes after eating a small plate of hot wings during happy hour.

Although heredity greatly determines your metabolic rate, another important factor that influences it is your body composition. If you're carrying around a lot of extra fat and not much muscle tissue, your metabolic rate will most likely be slow. Conversely, if you have little body fat and a high percentage of muscle, your metabolic rate will be much higher. As you can see, by increasing your body's percentage of muscle, your body will burn more calories throughout the day, whether you're working out or just kicking back.

Studies also show that your metabolism isn't so much influenced by *what* you eat, but rather by how *much* you eat. If you restrict your caloric intake too much, your metabolism will slow down in hopes of conserving energy. The kind of food you actually eat doesn't play much of a role, although, yes, I too have heard the rumors that eating foods such as hot chili peppers, spicy food, and curry can boost your metabolism. But studies show that eating all this spicy food would more likely play a role in boosting heartburn than speeding up your metabolism. My guess is that the reason people who eat a lot of spicy food may be thinner than those who don't is that they have to drink a lot of water in order to put out the fire they've ignited on their tongue. The water fills up their stomach; hence, they eat less food.

What it all boils down to is this: If you're looking for an excuse for being overweight, claiming to have a slow metabolism is a real winner. But if you're also looking for something to do about it, understanding your metabolic rate gives you the power to change things. The best thing you can do to speed up a slow metabolism is to steer clear of extreme diets that provide too few calories, and make sure that you incorporate exercise into your daily routine. Keep in mind that not all exercise is created equal. Sure, cardio work such as walking, bike riding, or spinning is great for your cardiovascular system and certainly burns extra calories in the short term. But the all-powerful metabolism-boosting form of exercise is weight training, in which you actually use added weight to tone muscles. That's because every pound of muscle that you add to your frame will cause it to burn approximately 43 extra calories a day. That may not sound like a lot on its own, but even if you can build just three extra pounds of muscle on your frame, you'd end up losing more than 13 pounds a year! So if you want to lose weight, get weights, and give your metabolism a good kick in the rear.

Time Isn't on My Side

Back in the old days when Howdy Doody dominated the airwaves and slingshots were an acceptable toy for kids to play with despite the fact that they knocked out the occasional eye, gender roles were clearly defined. Men worked at the office while the women stayed home all day cleaning the house, caring for the children, and sucking down a steady stream of tranquilizers. Back then, there was ample time to make slow-cooked meals and plenty of time to eat them around a family table.

But those days are over. Now the slow-cooked meals are replaced by greasy fast food, and slingshots are replaced by safety-approved toys that are so boring that kids have more fun playing with the boxes they came in. More often than not, both parents work outside the home, and the kids are busy with soccer practice, dance lessons, and so much homework that they actually have to carry it home in a wheeled suitcase. By the time parents and children arrive home at the end of the day, no one has the time to unwind, let alone fix a healthy, balanced meal. Instead, they tend to pick up dinner on the way home at a fast-food joint that serves food in a bucket. Your lack of free time thus becomes another wonderful excuse for your lack of a figure.

It doesn't have to be this way, though. Even with the busiest of schedules, there's still ample time to cook a low-calorie, healthy meal that you can make in less time than it takes to go through a crowded drive-through. In fact, I have a perfect solution for cooking fast in a fast-paced world. Its name is Crock-Pot (aka slow cooker).

The Crock-Pot is one of the best inventions of our times, along with shelf bras and ceramic flattening irons. The great thing about a slow cooker is that you throw all the ingredients into it in the morning, and by the time you arrive home at the end of a day, you're greeted by the smell of good old-fashioned home cooking. No matter what you put into this electric miracle, everything comes out tender and tasty. There's no need to sear your meat or sauté your vegetables ahead of time. And, best of all, there's only one nonstick pot to clean. If you don't have a slow cooker, I suggest that you head on down to your local discount store and get one. They're cheap to buy, easy to use, don't heat up your kitchen, and, might I say again, so easy to clean.

Most slow cookers come with a small recipe book included in the box, but there are also many great cookbooks that are geared toward Crock-Pot cooking. Almost all the recipes combine some sort of meat (you should use lean meats such as chicken and lean cuts of beef), some form of starch (which you can forgo if you don't want the extra carbs), and plenty of veggies. Toss in a few spices and a liquid of some kind, such as stock or wine, and you're ready to go! Here are a few delicious combinations:

- Chicken breasts, mushrooms, carrots, garlic, chicken broth, and sage
- Lean brisket, onions, potatoes, carrots, beef stock, red wine, and rosemary
- Pork loin, fennel, onions, red peppers, chicken stock, and apple cider vinegar

But man does not live by Crock-Pot cooking alone. Even though it's a wonderful cooking tool, you may want to supplement it with quick and easy recipes from books such as *30-Minute Meals* and *30-Minute Meals 2* by Rachael Ray. You may say that you don't even have a spare 30 minutes for cooking, but if you double the recipe, you can rationalize that it took only 15 minutes per meal. In fact, if you make thirty servings in one sitting, you'll get the time down to only one minute per! Now that's fast food!

Getting Older

Fact: As we age our face gets wrinkles, our hair turns gray, and the skin under our arms can hang so low that we could actually become airborne. In addition, as we get older, our bodies need less food in order to maintain their weight than they did before, and our desire to exercise gets tossed to the wayside, along with our old tube tops and painter's pants. Although these facts sound rather depressing, they give us a well-documented, medically valid reason for gaining weight that puts no blame on our lack of willpower whatsoever. So despite the fact that you may be depressed about turning forty, you're given the wonderful gift of a scientifically sound reason for your weight gain, as well as a new name for it: middle-age spread.

When we have a milestone birthday, whether it be thirty, forty, fifty, or some other age that is "scary" for us, we get nostalgic and think back to the innocent days of our youth. We remember the good old days, when we could eat Halloween candy without having to get it x-rayed first, stay out past dark without the fear of abduction, and best of all, eat anything we wanted to without ever getting fat. To paraphrase Dorothy when she was saying goodbye to the Scarecrow, "I'm going to miss that most of all."

The experts tell us that our bodies are at their peak of performance around the age of twenty-five But after that age, our metabolic rate decreases by about 2 to 8 percent each decade, forcing our bodies to slow down as fast as Jennifer Grey's career. This explains the mystery as to why you may eat the same amount of food as you did in the past, but keep on gaining weight.

It seems that the most significant time of weight gain in a woman's life starts around the age of forty. Studies show that at about this age, women gain an average of one pound a year. Not only does the weight go on at a faster rate than it did before, but the place where the weight is gained changes too. Before hitting forty, women store fat on their hips, butt, and thighs, but after forty, it tends to mass around the middle. This abdominal fat contributes to higher levels of cholesterol, higher blood fats, and higher blood pressure too. It seems that as we age, our once-shy and quiet fat develops the personality of Leona Helmsley.

Going through menopause is another a time of unexpected weight gain. It seems that along with dryness, bitchiness, and hot flashes comes the ability to pack on the pounds like Delta Burke during the *Designing Women* years. One of the reasons for this is that during menopause, our thyroid functions less effectively, making it easier to gain weight. Ironically, if you try to fight the fat by going on an extreme diet that severely cuts back on calories or carbohydrates, it tends to make matters even worse. And, according to some

> **❝** Now that I'm almost 50, I look at my body and I don't recognize it anymore. I used to have a really skinny waist but now I'm thick around the middle. Somehow I lost my waistline when I lost my ability to ovulate. **❞**
>
> —Sheila

studies, diets can also inhibit the production of sex hormones which, God knows, during menopause are in as short supply as rent-controlled apartments in New York City.

I know the facts seem depressing, but don't let them get you down. Just because you're going through "the change" doesn't mean that your fat cells have to go through it as well. The trick seems to be to stay ahead of the spread if you're young enough to catch it in time. Just by making a few simple changes to your diet, you can prevent this weight gain of one pound per year. Considering that one pound of fat equals 3,500 calories, all you have to do is reduce your annual caloric consumption by 3,500 per year, which translates to fewer than 10 calories a day. Sure, you could cut back on your food a little, but I've found an easier way. Laugh. Yes, laugh. Studies show that if you laugh out loud for about five minutes a day, you'll burn up to 10 calories. So, go ahead and listen to Howard Stern or stay up for Letterman's Top Ten. Or watch a *Seinfeld* marathon and fill your quota for the whole year. Laughter can not only lower your weight, but may also raise your spirits, which will come in handy when your sex drives plummets as low as Tom Cruise's approval rating after he jumped on Oprah's couch.

The Deviled Eggs Made Me Do It

If all else fails, you can actually blame your weight on the food itself. I know it seems like a stretch, but there have been many court cases where people have sued fast-food restaurants. They blame such places a McDonald's and Burger King because they serve up greasy, high-calorie, fattening food that they blame for their weight gain.

Although many people scoff at these cases, there is some validity to them. Today's food is far more fattening than in any other era in history. Never before has there been such a wide range of unhealthy and densely caloric foods, such as high-fructose corn syrup, bleached flour, and White Castle burgers. Also, today's marketing plays a role in obesity. In the early 1980s, the Reagan administration decided to do away with most regulations that restricted advertising to children. Because of this change, there was a tremendous increase in the number of commercials geared toward these young, impressionable tots, namely those for candy and fast food. As you know, children tend to want things they see on TV, thereby explaining the 1996 Tickle Me Elmo sensation.

Although I think blaming food manufacturers and fast-food franchises for your weight problem may be a stretch, it's totally relatable. Most of us get weak in the knees whenever we pass by Cinnabon at the food court. Our mouths

"I guarantee that if Sara Lee's father didn't have a gleam in his eye the night Sara was conceived, I'd be fifteen pounds lighter."

—Lisa

water when we smell the garlic rolls at our favorite Italian restaurant, and our tummies rumble whenever we get a whiff of a homemade waffle cone at an ice-cream store. I also know how much easier it is to blame others than it is to blame myself, which is why I'm convinced that my husband turns off the alarm in his sleep instead of entertaining the possibility that I could have forgotten to set it.

The trick to abstaining from life's little goodies is to prepare for them. As they say, strategy is stronger than willpower. Well, maybe "they" don't say that. I actually only heard that from one guy awhile back, but it stuck with me, so I thought it was worth mentioning. If you can't drive past your favorite doughnut shop without stopping in for a wake-up funnel cake, then take a different route to work. If you can't open your freezer without grabbing a frozen Milky Way bar that you put in there for a mother-in-law emergency, then stop buying them. As they say, "Out of sight, out of mind." This time, it really is "they" who said this, although "they" also said, "Absence makes the heart grow fonder," which is the totally opposite thing. I think "they" need to stop making up sayings after they've nipped at the brandy.

Look, I know that these ideas are much easier said than done. I know that, in reality, there may not be an alternate route to work, and there are probably other people living in your house who need that frozen Milky Way bar fix as much as you do. But maybe there's a compromise. Fast-food companies are actually changing their high-saturated-fat ways and now include healthy options on their menus, such as sliced fruit and salads with low-cal dressing. Food manufacturers are actually baking some of their popular snack foods instead of frying them, and even if they do fry them, they do so without the use of any trans fat. Maybe soon, there won't be any more cases of people suing fast-food chains because fast-food chains will only offer healthy meals. But until that day, don't sue any more restaurants, especially my Cinnabon place at the mall. A life without an occasional indulgence at Cinnabon is really a life not worth living!

Bad Health

Being in poor health may indeed make your life more challenging, but the good news is that it gives you the perfect excuse for rationalizing your weight. The truth is, there are several ailments that make adhering to a diet simply impossible. For instance, you could be allergic to a certain kind of food, like dairy or wheat, or you could have trouble digesting certain vegetables. But some of the biggest health problems that make dieting difficult are actually a by-product of being overweight in the first place. Sounds like a Catch-22, huh? Or maybe a Catch Type 2, since one of the most common symptoms of being overweight is type 2 diabetes.

Although anyone could be a candidate for getting type 2 diabetes, you're twice as likely to have it if you're overweight. If you're diagnosed with diabetes, you'll be advised to follow a healthy diet that's no doubt the complete opposite of what you're used to eating. Because of this, patients tend to follow one of two distinct paths. One is to follow the diet to the letter, like my sister-in-law, Pam. She eats at regular intervals, brings special food with her to functions, and weeps every Halloween for the beloved bite-sized candies that she'll forever mourn. The other path is to ignore the diet completely, like my good friend Cindy. Whenever I meet Cindy for coffee, she chows down on her glazed maple bar with one hand and shoots herself up with insulin with the other. It really is nice to have a friend like Cindy. Not because our get-togethers are so pleasant (it's hard having a deep conversation when someone is searching for a body part that's not black-and-blue from previous injections), but because it's comforting to know that if I ever need fertility drugs, she's an excellent person to give them to me.

Being a diabetic greatly restricts the kinds of diets that you can actually go on. Because a diabetic needs to keep her blood sugar level steady, she can't go on one of those trendy cleansing diets where you eat nothing but water and cayenne pepper. Also, Atkins and other similar, low-carb diets are out because a diabetic needs carbohydrates. Sure, eating a healthy diet full of fruits, vegetables, and lean proteins is ideal, but it's not nearly as much fun as following the trendy diet that gave Jessica Simpson her Daisy Duke butt.

Gout is another physical condition that can be caused by being overweight. Gout is incredibly painful and usually affects the joint in the big toe. Like type 2 diabetes, the best cure would be to lose weight, but having the condition makes dieting more difficult. For instance, if you have gout, you shouldn't go on a high-protein, low-carbohydrate diet, for it could easily make the condition worse.

Although exercise is a great way to lose weight, being overweight makes exercise much more painful than it is for a thinner person. Carrying around an extra 50 pounds or so is like walking around with a golden retriever. It's enough of a workout just walking to the end of your driveway for the paper, let alone doing a half hour on a treadmill. When you're heavy, you don't have the endurance of a lean, mean wrecking machine. Also, working out when you're over-weight can be very hard on your back and knees.

Between you and me, being overweight doesn't mean that getting in shape can't be done. Rather, it means that it has to be done slowly. But, duh, you don't really need me to tell you that. Just look for exercises that are very low impact, such as walking, swimming, dancing, or using an elliptical machine. Look for gyms like Curves that cater more toward heavier people, or any knockoff of this fran-chise that may have surfaced in your area. Gyms like these are not so intimidating to join. As they say (there "they" are again!), where there's a will, there's a way. And if you don't want your will to be read in the near future, you'd better find a way to exercise.

Of course, as with any exercise program, you should check with your doctor before you begin. I say this not because I would do this myself, but because I don't want any one of you out there to sprain an ankle and come after me. There may be one or two of you who are bitter about an unsuccess-ful McDonald's lawsuit and figure I'd be an easier target.

Money Is the Root of All Evil Weight Gain

When it comes to excuses, you can always give the poverty excuse a try. What it all boils down to is that people blame the fact that they're overweight on the fact that they don't make enough money to afford to eat right. Now you gotta admit, this excuse may seem a bit far-fetched, but it's pretty creative! It's the Tim Burton of excuses. The truth, though, is that being obese is not only bad for your health, it's bad for your wealth as well.

Anybody who's ever bought food knows that food that's good for you tends to be more expensive than food that's not. Fresh vegetables cost more than canned. Fresh fish costs more than the frozen breaded version found in stick form. And while I agree that the high price of food can take a big bite out of any paycheck and may seem like a valid excuse for being heavy, the truth is that the difference in the cost of food is far outweighed by the hidden expenses that come along with being overweight.

When looking at the expenses of being heavy, one needs to see the whole picture. For instance, clothing tends to be more costly when you're restricted to buying it at plus-size shops. You may also want additional items, including slimming girdles, jackets that conceal your trouble zones, designer clothing with deflecting patterns, and various accessories, such as pins or scarves, to distract the eye. Also, if you're overweight, you're more likely to have health problems that translate into higher doctor bills, more medications, and a more costly life-insurance premium. Bryan Krupin, from Gilbert-Krupin Insurance, estimates that an overweight person may spend an average of 75 percent more on life insurance depending on age and degree of extra weight. In addition, being overweight may cause you to miss more work because of health problems, translating to less money in your paycheck if you're paid by the hour. You may also need to buy sturdier furniture, which costs more than the standard items, or even have to buy two airplane tickets for your next trip. There's even one final expense that I'll bet you haven't thought of: It can be twice as costly to buy an oversized coffin than to get one that's standard size. If the thought of all the money you'll lose by being overweight isn't enough to make you have mackerel instead of mac & cheese tonight, I don't know what is.

Aside from these extraneous expenses, it's just a fact that a person who's heavy simply eats more food than a person who's thin. And the cost of all that extra junk can easily offset the cost of buying fresh, wholesome food in the first place. So, if you're blaming your full figure on the fact that you have an empty wallet, realize that you're not taking all the costs into account. Besides, the best way to save money on food is to eat at home instead of going out. Studies show that 46 percent of the family food budget is spent on meals outside the home. And within that, 34 percent is spent on fast-food places. So as you can see, an ounce of preventing yourself from buying junk food is worth a pound of fat that you'll gain if you don't.

Dem Bones

People often rationalize the fact that they weigh a lot by saying they're just big boned. In fact, it's fair to say that people use this excuse more than all the others combined. And why shouldn't they? The size of a person's bones can directly affect a person's weight (although granted, some would have to have bones the size of a *T. rex's* to rationalize their weight).

Everyone knows that heredity plays a big part in body weight, and that if someone comes from a "big boned" family, they're more likely to be heavy. Statistics say that if both parents are obese, their children are actually 80 percent more likely to become obese as well. If only one parent is obese,

> **"** When I was growing up, we'd always have a big Sunday night dinner and all the kids would have a contest to see who could eat the most rolls. I always seemed to be the winner, and to this day I still carry around the prize of the rolls of fat I gained. **"**
>
> —Susanna

the risk drops to 40 percent. And if neither parent is obese, then the likelihood plummets to only a 15 percent chance. But statistics don't always tell the whole story. For instance, some people theorize that the reason obesity runs in families has more to do with circumstance than it does with genetics. When their parents are overweight, children are much more likely to sit down to a dinner of chicken-fried steak than a light poached salmon salad. Also, children whose parents are heavy may lead a far more sedentary lifestyle than those whose parents aren't. Their weekends may revolve around ordering pizza and renting videos as opposed to going on a family bike ride.

The fact is that obesity is a relatively new phenomenon, and it seems to be getting worse every year. Back in 1976, only 14 percent of the population was obese, but in the year 2000, that number climbed to 30 percent. If a person's body weight is really determined by heredity alone, then obesity rates would have stayed constant. If you deep-down feel that you're locked into a big body because of your big family, take a look at some old family photographs of your grandparents and your great-grandparents. You may find that instead of seeing people with extra chins and spare tires, you'll see a bunch of relatives of normal weight staring back at you in that disturbing way they did in the days of black-and-white photography.

Maybe after seeing those pictures, you'll feel relieved and inspired to lose some weight. Maybe you'll also see that your love of all things pork may play as big a role in your weight as do family genetics. Sure, you can't do much to change the size of your nose or the size of your feet by sheer willpower and motivation, but you certainly can alter the size of your ass.

Diets Don't Work

One of the most valid excuses that you can give is that you've gone on every diet that's out there and that the diets just didn't work. Either you weren't able to lose any weight or, if you did, you ended up gaining back more weight than you lost in the first place. In most cases you're right in thinking that diets are about as effective as FEMA was during Hurricane Katrina. The biggest culprits have got to be fad diets that come and go like hem lengths. For instance, who can forget past diets like the popcorn diet, the chocolate diet, or the grapefruit diet? And who can say that in the future, someone won't mock today's trends, such as Atkins or the Zone? Popular diet books tend to have a shelf life of just a few years, and a tad longer if they've been mentioned on *The View*. These trendy diets are the shoulder pads, corky shoes, and stirrup pants of the diet world.

The reason people have trouble following a certain diet is that they fall victim to the hype. They've seen the before-and-after shots. They've heard the testimonials. And they believe it when the book tells them that the diet is so easy to follow. They see the plan laid out before them in black and white, and understand the author's logic about how they can eat less and never be hungry. But then they start the diet and realize that they've been betrayed when it takes them on the same hellish ride as all the others before it. And just as with all the other diets, people end up at the exact same place: the closest Wetzel's Pretzels stand for a Cin-A-Yum pretzel.

There are plenty of experts who would agree that diets don't work. They proclaim that the only true way to lose weight is to stop dieting altogether. It's only then that our bodies can adjust to normal eating and begin to lose weight permanently. These so-called experts preach that the only way to find permanent weight loss is to stop trying. But keep in mind that it's experts who also tell us that the only way to find true love is to stop looking. Personally, I'm not such a fan of either of these methods. I believe that some things worth getting are worth putting effort into. I know that I've never lost weight by not trying, and I have never been able to find my lost keys without looking for them. It's only after an exhausting room-by-room search that I finally find them among my daughter's other "treasures," like her pen cap collection and my old bra, which she uses as a hammock for her Polly Pocket dolls.

Less Believable Excuses

If you're not too fond of any of the excuses I just mentioned, maybe you need a list that's a bit more eclectic. Here are a few more excuses that may not be as believable, but are at least more creative:

- You got cast for the lead in Bridget Jones III and you need to plump up.
- The way you stand now, you don't weigh enough to close your overstuffed suitcase when you sit on it.
- You're hoping to be a model in the next Dove soap magazine spread.
- You're in training for next year's pie-eating contest.
- Tragically, you were born without that certain brain chemical that tells you when you're full.

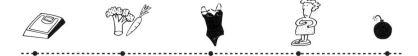

chapter eight

keeping the weight off

With most challenges in life, once you achieve your goal, the challenge is over. Once you get your college degree, you don't have to take any more classes. Once you get a job, you don't have to pound any more pavement. And once you deliver your baby, you don't have to push out anything else (except for that nasty placenta, which really is a joy-kill). But with weight loss, the situation is far different. Once you reach your goal weight, the challenge is only half over. That's because now comes the incredibly difficult task of actually keeping the weight off, which may be just as tough, or even tougher, than losing it in the first place.

I consider myself to be an excellent dieter. In fact, I've lost a total of 182 pounds over my lifetime. By all measures, I should be the size of a CornNut. But obviously, I have quite a bit of trouble actually keeping the weight off. If you have any experience in the dieting milieu, then you know exactly from where I speak. You'd think that after all the long months of dieting, you'd have learned some healthy eating habits that would prohibit you from gaining the weight back. You'd think that your new slender frame would once and for all stop its intense craving for guacamole. And you'd think that after all these years, people would stop believing that a certain Beatles song played backward says "Paul is Dead." But in all these cases, you'd be absolutely wrong.

The cold, hard truth is that it's much easier to gain the weight back than it is to lose it in the first place. And so much more fun too! For instance, it can easily take me a week to lose two pounds, but only one meal at TGI Friday's to gain it all back. So heed my warning: If you've reached your goal weight and are tempted to go off track, even for just a day, realize that going back to your old eating habits is as dangerous as setting a small brush fire, which can quickly spread to your upper arms and outer thighs.

I know all too well that once you regain a certain amount of weight, you're at a crucial fork in the road. You can either find the strength to start back up on your diet, or just say the hell with it and eat yourself back to the weight you were when you first started. And we both know that the chances of going back on your diet are the same as letting your son have a sleepover at Neverland Ranch.

So if you're having a hard time keeping off the weight that you've struggled so hard to lose, read on. Here you'll discover some of the most common reasons a dieter can be tempted to overindulge. Hopefully, you can recognize yourself in one of them, realize how common it is, and stop yourself before you dive face first into that bowl of guacamole. Yes, now that you're down to your fighting weight, get back in the ring and remember the first rule of dieting rebound: No gaining weight below the belt!

Self-Sabatoge

I'm my worst enemy when it comes to things like critiquing my own work and judging the size of a nasty pimple that's grown on my nose. And I'm also my own worst enemy when it comes to keeping my new figure after dieting. For some mysterious reason that I can never understand despite years of soul searching and countless hours listening to Dr. Laura, I quickly regain all the weight after I finish a diet. I'd understand my behavior if I was suddenly put under a lot of stress, or my fantasy about taking a bath in a tub full of Nutter Butter bars had finally come true. But alas, neither of these scenarios has occurred, and I'm left feeling as confused as ever as to why I binge back to my bulbous state.

Maybe you're like me and have trouble maintaining your new weight, and have disturbing fantasies about peanutty-flavored cookies. You too may have tried to analyze the reason for your weakness, but the truth is that there can be several reasons why you're a self-sabatoger. We women are complicated beings, which explains our frequent mood swings and why we buy organic food yet don't think twice about having our faces injected with Botox. We're like an estrogen-filled onion with many layers of skin, all of which we like to have exfoliated and moisturized with expensive imported lotions. This means that there can be many reasons for self-sabatoge, all of which are quite common among us womenfolk.

For one thing, we may not feel comfortable in our new, leaner skin. We feel self-conscious when men compliment us or whistle at us as we stroll past. We may be afraid of what our new skinny future could bring. What if our new looks and confidence finally land us that great boyfriend we've always dreamed of, or that wonderful job we aspire to have? For years that's what we've yearned for, and now that it's within reach, it can be a very scary proposition. In fact, it may scare us so much that we retreat back into our old comfortable world filled with overalls and elastic waistbands.

When we lose weight, we're left with nothing to hide behind. Before, we could blame all of our unhappiness on our hefty calves: *Why would someone invite me to their party when they know I'd eat all of the appetizers?* But then once we're finally thin and we *still* don't get invited to parties, we have no alternative but to blame ourselves. The fact remains that no matter how much fat someone loses, she can still be the same self-centered bitch she always was, only she looks better in a clingy knit dress. When faced with that reality, many people seek out head cheese instead of a head shrinker.

Another reason women sabotage themselves is that they don't think they deserve to be thin. As you know, women are not big on feeling deserving. We think that being slender and attractive are traits only suited for movie stars and members of the Hilton family. Instead, we're big on feeling unworthy. It's one of our most self-destructive traits, along with our tendency to be clingy after having sex with someone for the first time.

I'm hoping that, now that you can see some of the silly reasons behind self-sabotage, you'll be able to stop yourself dead in your tracks before you've done too much damage to your weight-loss success. And if it turns out that you are indeed self-sabotaging yourself, take comfort in the fact that you're not alone. Being a self-sabotageur is more common than sitting next to a mouth-breather at a crowded movie theater.

Friends and Family

Friends and family may be great when you're looking for love, support, and donations to your kid's walk-a-thon fundraiser at school, but you shouldn't necessarily turn to them for help when you need support on your diet. In fact, these people may turn out to be the worst sabotagers of them all.

Oftentimes, the most common offender turns out to be the one you promised to love, honor, and pamper when he's sick till death do you part. Now that you're looking all hot and sexy, it's your husband who may start to feel insecure. Sure, part of him really likes the new you, especially the part of himself that he refers to as "Big Johnny," but the rest of him may have more conflicted feelings. He may feel jealous of the way other men look at you. He may worry that you'll find someone else you're more attracted to. Yes, now that you've trimmed down, you walk a fine line between turning him on and turning him off.

Your family may not be too pleased about the fact that there's less of you to love either. For one thing, they may be jealous that you've managed to do something that they could never find the willpower to do. They also may not feel comfortable with you in your new role as the skinny one in the family. If you have sisters, they may be the worst offenders of all, because sisters tend to be quite competitive with one another. I know that for my whole life, my sister compared everything from our bellybuttons to our arm hair in a lame-ass attempt to make herself feel superior. *Arm hair*, for heaven's sake!

But family members aren't the only ones who might have a problem with the new you. Friends may feel a bit spiteful as well. If you and your friends used to spend a lot of

66 Every time I go on a diet, my coworkers insist on going to

lunch at a place that only serves greasy food I'm not able to

eat. I don't want to be a problem so I go with them and end up

going off my diet. Sure I could change jobs and lose weight, but

I'd also lose my great insurance and matching 401(k) plan.**99**

—Janie

time complaining about your weight issues, you'll now have to find something else to talk about. Also, your friends may have relied on you to be the fourth at the "buy three, get one free" deal at Nougat World. Or maybe they liked having you in their circle of friends because you used to make them look thin by comparison.

Because those around you may have problems with the new thinner you, they may actually set you up for failure. They might bring over goodies and tell you it's okay to have just a few. They may tell you horror stories about people who were on the same diet as you and gained back all their weight in a week. Or they may enroll you in the "cake of the month" club.

It doesn't take long to realize that some of your relationships may be more detrimental to your diet than that big tub of licorice in the snack room. It seems that in addition to gaining more willpower around sweets, you also have to gain a strong backbone around sabotagers. You have to be able to say no to their bad will without the fear of upsetting them, because they certainly don't have your best interests at heart. You have to push away their temptations, and cancel your membership to that cake of the month club, which is a total killer, because there really is nothing better than cake. You need to realize that if you do upset your sabotagers and, in turn, lose them, there's really no healthier form of weight loss you can have!

The Good Old Days

Some people are nostalgic for the "good old days." The days when you could call a company and actually speak to a real person instead of a computer operator. The days when you could go through an airport security line without having to expose your undarned socks. And the days when you could polish off a pint of ice cream without guilt. But now those days are over, and if you want to be able to fit into your "slim" jeans instead of your "relaxed fit," you believe you'll have to abstain from pigging out for the rest of your life. And that thought scares you more than the first time you saw male genitalia.

I too would panic if I felt that I'd have to give up my guilty pleasures for the rest of my life. Some of my fondest memories are those I've shared with my good friends Ben & Jerry. I've shed more tears with my gal pal Sara Lee than with some of my closest friends. And a world without Little Debbie is not a world that I want to be a part of. Besides, how can I possibly be expected to watch a movie without a bag of bulk candy on my lap that contains the perfect balance of Reese's Pieces, malted milk balls, and red Swedish Fish? Just the thought of having to give up these pleasures forever so I can look good in a midriff-baring top makes me want to run to the nearest In-N-Out Burger for a double-double-dose of reality.

I know what you're thinking. You think that I should still be able to have a cookie from time to time. And although you're right in theory, there is no such thing as "just a cookie" with me. When it comes to sugary snacks, I'm an all-or-nothing kind of gal. I'm jealous of those people who can have just one piece of candy and call it a day. Those are the kind of people who will most likely be able to keep their weight off for their whole lives. They believe in things like moderation and single-size servings, and can actually live what they preach. Me, I believe that a life devoid of creamy centers is really no life at all.

If you're having a hard time coming to grips with the fact that you can't return to your old gluttonous eating habits, you're not alone. It's a scary world out there without your old pals around to comfort you. And the thought of being alone out there makes you want to seek comfort in the arms of your friend Colonel Sanders. But here are some tips in hopes that you can have your cake and eat it on occasion to:

If you want to snack on a few cookies, take one or two out of the bag and put them on a plate. As we all know, if you have the bag in front of you, it's all over. Also, once you're done taking the cookies out of the bag, toss it up on a really high shelf where it's out of reach without the use of a step-ladder. Hopefully your laziness will be stronger than your snack attack.

When you're at a restaurant and you want dessert, order what you want, take one bite out of it, and pour a bunch of salt on the rest. Unless you've ordered a hot pretzel, it'll be totally inedible.

If you're at a party with a friend, promise her that if you overindulge, you'll give her $100. And you can't back out of the deal.

If you can't resist that bulk candy display (and God knows I can't), have a neutral party fill your candy bowl with just a few tastes of what you want. I also find that a jawbreaker is a good sugary treat to bring to the theater because it takes a long time to eat. Of course you'll make up the time when you need to have the resulting cavities filled, but in the meantime, you're better off in terms of calories.

Buy prepackaged treats that won't do much damage to your diet, such as Nabisco's 100 Calorie Packs of Oreo Crisps or chocolate chip cookies or one of a wide variety of crackers. Pop Secret also has a line of 100-calorie bags of popcorn, called 100 Calorie Pop, which are great to snack on in front of the TV or to take with you to a movie so you can resist the fattening, overpriced movie popcorn.

Chew the Fat

Most times you know when you're cheating on your diet. You'll order a plate of onion rings knowing full well that it's breaking every diet rule in the book. But other times you may think that what you're eating is actually healthy, when in reality, it may have even more fat and calories than the onion rings. So, before you accidentally jeopardize your weight loss with something that you think is diet cuisine, memorize this list of some of the biggest culprits when it comes to food with the most hidden calories:

1. Muffins: Most regular-sized muffins have as much fat as a slice of cake. You can have a mini-size muffin if you'd like, but sometimes it's just enough to make you mad that you're not eating a full-sized muffin.

2. Granola: This popular food of the hippie generation is now popular with today's overweight generation of people who are just plain hippy. That's because this so-called health food is full of fat and calories.

3. Salad dressing: Oily or creamy dressings have so many calories that you'd be better off if you just mixed those healthy greens with pie filling.

4. Chicken sandwiches at fast-food restaurants: I know it may sound better to order a chicken sandwich than a burger, but oftentimes there's not much difference in the calories. Between the crispy crust and the mayonnaise, there's as much fat content as there is at a *What's Happening!!* reunion show.

5. Protein bars: Unless you're going to run a marathon, I'd steer clear of this type of food, which has enough calories to sustain a third-world country.

6. Tuna and egg salad sandwiches: Be careful of sandwiches that are laden with mayonnaise, such as tuna, egg, chicken, seafood, or ham salad sandwiches. Eaten alone, these foods can be quite healthy, but with all that fat mixed in, they're as bad for your health as a nerve-wracking blind date.

7. Fat-free desserts: Just because something is free of fat doesn't mean that it's free of calories—that is, unless it's fat free AND calorie free, in which case, you're simply eating air.

8. Movie popcorn: There's as much fat in a big bucket of popcorn as there is in six hamburgers, and that's

without pumping on that imitation butter flavor, which can double as car grease!

The Whac-a-Mole Syndrome

One of the main reasons that losing weight is only half of a weight-loss success story is because of the numerous events that center around food, or at least where you center around the food table. One by one, these parties filled with platters of savory sensations and sinful sweets try to eat away at your willpower, which in turn, eats away at your diet success. Each of these events is like a chocolate-covered Whac-a-Mole game trying to pound you over the head until you're too weak to say no to temptation.

Of course, we can avoid these temptations by simply avoiding places where food will be served. Sure, I know that food is everywhere, but there's a difference between going to an afternoon tea party that serves miniature watercress sandwiches and taking a weeklong cruise, which is really just a giant buoyant buffet table.

It's not just the official holiday season, the most wonderfully fattening time of the year, that causes the problems. There are so many occasions that focus on food scattered throughout the year, and they are the demise of many diet success stories. If you have the willpower, strength, and stamina to endure just one of them, there's another one waiting right around the bend to pound you over the head yet again. If you can make it through a New Year's Eve party without indulging in too much champagne and hors d'oeuvres, then comes Valentine's Day with its heart-shaped boxes of cream-filled chocolates, which are the Saddam

Hussein of any diet. Then comes the stuffed cabbage and green beer of St. Patrick's Day, and the chocolate eggs and Marshmallow Peeps of Easter. Butted smack dab up against that is the BBQ bonanza of Memorial Day, the fun and fattening Fourth of July, the block party sensation of summer vacation, and the luscious Labor Day weekend.

As if that's not enough to loosen your belt, don't forget that sprinkled in between those events are numerous birthdays, weddings, baptisms, bar mitzvahs, anniversaries, and graduations, all of which are celebrated by stuffing our faces. Just think of each year as 365 days to indulge!

Unless you have the willpower of a priest at a nude beach, chances are strong that you'll nibble on a box of Valentine's treats, indulge in ample amounts of BBQ ribs, and bite off the heads of one too many Marshmallow Peeps. Little by little, pound by pound, the weight begins to rebuild itself like a city after a war.

The trick, of course, is to learn to celebrate the event itself, and not the big bowl of Chex Party Mix that is *at* the event. Of course, that's a very difficult trick indeed, and harder to master than the one where you touch your tongue to your nose. But if you can perfect it, you will stand a far better chance of keeping the pounds at bay. And if you can perfect the tongue-to-nose trick, you can make a room full of men stare at you with a dumb expression on their faces.

So the next time you're at a wedding, hit the dance floor instead of the dessert table. When you're at your neighbor's barbecue, hit the pool instead of the pork ribs. And when you're at your husband's company cocktail party, well, then, just go ahead and indulge, because there's really no other way to get through those horrible things if you don't.

Yo-Yo Dieting

A very common syndrome that occurs among dieters is to lose weight on a diet, gain it all back again, lose it once more, and then gain it back yet another time. This pattern tends to continue from diet to diet, year after year. This form of dieting is called "yo-yo" dieting, and it happens more often than getting stuck in the slow line at the grocery store.

I consider myself quite the expert on the subject of yo-yo dieting. In fact, I'm the yo-yo Ma of the diet world. Fortunately, there is no reason to believe that you'll have any problems achieving success with a diet just because your weight fluctuated as often as the price of gold on other diets. If you do some hard-core research, like I did (which consisted of clicking onto a few impressive-looking Web sites), you'll find that several experts agree that yo-yo dieting doesn't alter your metabolism, doesn't create any additional health concerns other than those caused by being overweight, and except for extreme dieting or for those who've gained back a lot more weight than they've lost, shouldn't leave you with any less muscle mass or additional fat cells.

That said, yo-yo dieting certainly isn't the best method of weight control either. The secret to avoiding yo-yo dieting is to go only on a diet that you can stick to once the diet is over. If you can't start your morning without a toasted onion bagel, then the Atkins diet might not make the most sense for you. If your budget is limited, avoid diets that require a pricey membership fee or expensive prepackaged food. And if you never did well with ratios in math class, I'd steer clear of the Zone. Instead, you should choose a diet that fits your lifestyle; one that will teach you how to eat right, instead of one that will only teach you how to eat right now.

For instance, if you went on Jenny Craig or NutriSystem, you may have lost a lot of weight, but all you learned about low-calorie food was how to order it on the company's Web site. You didn't learn how to cook healthy meals or how to make good selections at restaurants. So once you got off of the diet, you were like a released prisoner without the skills that are learned at a halfway house. You're out of control when faced with real food that doesn't come in a box, so every meal turns out to be one big fattening conjugal visit.

Even though yo-yo dieting can get frustrating, try not to get discouraged. Just because you gained back the weight you lost doesn't mean you won't succeed in keeping it off the next time around. I've heard it said that it takes smokers an average of seven times to quit smoking before they finally stop. Maybe it will take you seven times to go on a diet before you find one that works. Or maybe it'll take you four times or twenty-four. Who knows? All I know is that you shouldn't stop trying. After all, I dated dozens of guys until I finally found one that was kind and reliable, and didn't steal my wallet when I was out of the room. Just remember, when you're ready to start your next diet, choose one that has basic guidelines you can follow for the rest of your life. To paraphrase an old adage, "Give a person a fish and he'll eat right for a day. Teach a person to make steamed fish with a soy ginger glaze, and he'll eat right for a lifetime."

The Best Things to Do If You
See the Weight Creeping Back

If you notice that your fingers have been dipping into that jar of peanut butter too often, or that you've indulged in one too many jelly doughnuts from the office lunchroom, it's not too late to stop your snacking and get back on track. What you need is a little push in order to find the strength to push away all the junk food that seems to be everywhere. Here are some ideas to help you get back on track.

1. Wear the jeans that you were finally able to fit into again, which are now becoming just a bit snug. Every time you sit down and you feel the tightness around your upper thigh area, it will be a constant reminder that you need to watch what you eat!

2. Exercise. Oftentimes, when you start to cheat on your diet, you tend to stop working out. But exercise will lift your spirits by filling you with endorphins and will keep you far away from temptation (unless, of course, your idea of lifting weights is raising a Philly cheese steak up to your mouth).

3. Give yourself an extra boost of motivation. Look at yourself naked in the mirror; put on a great top that's just a little bit small for you; or, better yet, tell your boyfriend that when you see him this weekend, you're going to make love to him with the lights on. Yeah, that oughtta do it!

Not So Great Expectations

Another reason people have a hard time keeping the weight off after going on a diet is that the diet didn't give them the results they were looking for. Sure, they may be able to slip into that slip dress they haven't been able to slip into for a while, but that's about it. Losing weight didn't give them more friends or a better job or a steamier love life. It didn't make them feel more comfortable at parties or better equipped to handle disappointments. It didn't give them inner strength or make them become more generous and less cynical. After all the hardship they endured to get to their goal weight, the only thing they really changed about themselves was their percentage of body fat.

For instance, if you overate because you lacked intimacy in your marriage, that lack may always be there no matter which dress size you can fit into. If you overate to help fill the void created by a lack of love when you were young, you'll still feel the void. Overall, a diet is only capable of correcting some of your physical flaws. It's not capable of correcting your character flaws as well.

Dr. Phil is a big advocate of this belief system. In fact, his popular book *The Ultimate Weight Solution* focuses on the importance of uncovering the reason that someone overeats in the first place. It's only *after* solving these problems that a person can finally begin to lose weight permanently. Don't get me wrong. I don't always believe that Dr. Phil can solve someone's lifelong crisis in between commercial breaks, but I do agree with him that people overeat due to some deep-rooted problem, and not just because of some deep-dish pizza.

❝I fought my weight for years and finally realized that I overate because I was jealous of my thin sister, since she got all the attention. I figured this out when she gained almost sixty pounds when she was pregnant with her twins and was never thin again.❞

—Daniela

So, if you went on a diet hoping that your life would be different, you may be disappointed. Sure, losing weight can give you more confidence and a better body image, but looking smashing in a backless dress isn't the key to happiness that some people believe it to be. Diets do shed pounds, but not the underlying problems.

To Gain or Not to Gain? Here Are Some Questions

Some people have a greater advantage than others when faced with certain challenges in life. Some people are born as natural athletes. Others have more brain power than brawn. Still others are better suited to keeping their weight off after going on a diet. They seem to have more determination. They seem to have more incentive. And they seem to be able to pass by a platter of crab cakes and just say no.

If you're curious to find out whether you have what it takes to keep off unwanted pounds, take the following quiz.

1. Can you watch a late-night pizza commercial without running over and licking the screen?
2. Can you see a toddler eating an ice-cream cone without fighting the urge to rip it out of its itty-bitty hand?
3. Does your stomach still growl in between meals with the intensity of one of those Jaws of Life machines?
4. Can you watch a woman breastfeeding her newborn without getting a craving for Dairy Queen?
5. Can you go to a cocktail party without eating a plate of cocktail franks?

6. Are you thinking about marrying your boyfriend just so you can eat cake in a room full of people without being judged?

Don't worry if you failed the test. As you may have guessed, it doesn't have any scientific basis or any controlled group study. It isn't even written by a weight-loss expert. In fact, I made it up myself just for laughs. But I do believe that there is some truth behind the theory that your eating pattern must change in order to keep the unwanted pounds from creeping back. If they do, you may be on your way back to South Beach once again.

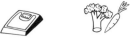

chapter nine

it's not over until the
fat lady manages to drop
those last ten pounds

This part of the book is rather tricky for me to write. I like happy endings—and not every diet has a happy ending. Sure, there are some of you out there who have conquered your cravings and triumphed over temptations, and were able to lose the weight that you set out to lose. Maybe you overcame some past trauma, or maybe you found the courage to end your relationship with Nutella, or maybe you simply switched to Diet Coke and called it a day. But whatever changes you made, you managed to beat the battle of the bulge, and I sincerely congratulate you!

Now, there's a whole new world of experiences awaiting you. You can have a stressful day and not turn to something glazed to make you feel better. You can go to your step class and not have to be in the back of the room so you can sneak out early without the instructor noticing. You can walk past a mirror and actually admire the reflection staring back at you. You can go to a party without spending the evening in front of the artichoke dip. And you can have sex without the fear of cutting a big one right in the middle of the act the way you used to do after eating four chili cheese dogs for dinner.

For the first time in a long time, a sweet summer peach actually sounds like a great way to end a meal. You eat five servings of fruits and vegetables just like the food pyramid recommends without even trying. You say no to junk and yes to heart-healthy food. Finally you feel good about yourself, and the owners of your local "All You Can Eat" buffet feel good about you too. That's because they're now able to make a profit off of you instead of losing their shirt every time you walk through their door!

But statistics show that there are many more of you who did not get to your goal weight. Even if you did, you ended up gaining the weight back again, and maybe even more. In fact, a 1994 report published by the National Academy of Sciences says that the average dieter regains two-thirds of the weight back within one year, and almost all of it within five. I don't say this to depress you. I say it so that if you weren't a big loser, you should take comfort in the fact that you're not alone.

As you know, losing weight is a very hard thing to do. One reason for this is the belief that our bodies have a natural "set point," a weight that they strive to attain. Whenever we diet, our metabolism slows down so that it won't lose this precious cargo. Soon, the hunger and cravings begin and the willpower fades, making it nearly impossible to resist temptation. If you ignore these warnings and continue to diet, your metabolism may slow down even further and fight back with a vengeance. You'll start to feel cold. You won't have much energy. You may even skip periods, which is nature's way of telling you that your body would have a hard time sustaining a pregnancy when its food supply is so low. As you can see, your body is quite a worthy opponent that plans its next move as adeptly as Bobby Fischer.

Even if you didn't win over your opponent this time, you shouldn't feel like a failure. Practice does indeed make perfect, and maybe on your next round, your diet strategy will prevail. Until that time, there are ways to look thinner, which we'll discuss in this section. Some of these methods involve a scalpel, while others merely involve a new pair of shoes. And of course, there is another option for dealing with your weight. It's called acceptance, which guarantees that you'll live happily every after no matter what the scale says. So even though this final chapter of the book may not be entirely optimistic, at least it makes me happy, because I've written just about everything I know about dieting!

Dress to Compress

Even if you have dropped a whole lotta weight, you may be struggling to lose those last ten pounds. For some unknown reason, the last ten tend to cling to you harder than a shy child on the first day of kindergarten. If you know a few handy-dandy secrets, you can hide those extra pounds until you find the inner strength to lose them, or enough duct tape to seal your mouth shut. Here are some of the best ways to camouflage those last, determined pounds:

Invest in a good bra. If you're a woman who has an ample bosom, it's crucial to keep those puppies lifted high and mighty. If they're dangling down around your waistline, they're going to bring the rest of you down with them. Go to a lingerie department and make sure that you ask a trained professional to measure you for size. Chances are high that you've been wearing the wrong size bra for years. The sign of a good bra is that it lifts your breasts high enough that they fall just between your shoulder and your elbow. If you want to look smaller, ask the saleslady to show you a minimizing bra. Sure, it may take some of the gleam out of your lover's eye, but it'll take the pounds off as well.

Buy yourself a girdle. Again, go to a good lingerie shop and ask for some assistance. These days, the racks are full of full-figure foundations that can flatten your stomach, lift up your ass, shrink down your thighs, and accomplish things that only a time machine can do.

Dress for your type. If you have a thicker waist, avoid tops that end at your midline. Instead, buy the ones that are long and loose in order to hide your midriff. If saddlebags are your problem, an A-line skirt is the answer. If you have large breasts, buy scoop necks instead of V-necks, which draw attention to your cleavage. The idea is to distract the eye away from your trouble zones. Also, if you're trying on pants and you're in between sizes, buy the larger of the two. I know we're all obsessed with fitting into the smallest size possible, but the looseness of the fabric in the larger size will actually make you look slimmer.

Wear clothes that are the same color. This can be either a dress that's all one color or pants and a top that are the same color. When you dress in this monochromatic style, you trick the eye into thinking that you're longer and leaner than you actually are.

If you have thick, curly hair, you may want to consider wearing it straight. Long, straight hair makes your face look longer and leaner than it does if you wear your hair thick and curly. There are amazing new products on the market these days that make it easy to get that sleek, flat look. There are frizz-reducer sprays and silicone lotions, and best of all, ceramic straightening irons that leave your hair as flat as Roseanne Barr's voice.

Accessories count. Instead of stud earrings, wear long dangly ones. Instead of a short scarf tied around your neck, wear one that's long. Instead of wearing flats, wear heels. Do anything that will elongate your look.

Listen to your mother and stand up straight! If you slouch, stick your shoulders back. If you have a swayback, pull your stomach in. Pretend that you're a marionette, with a string that goes from the bottom of your feet through the top of your head, and that some puppeteer is pulling you up. I know it feels uncomfortable, but check your new look in the mirror. I think you'll agree that by simply standing up straight, you'll look ten pounds lighter.

If you're having your photo taken, pose like a celebrity. Look in any fashion magazine and you'll notice that all the models turn their lower half to the side while their upper half faces toward the camera. Then they point one foot straight ahead and the other to the side. Once you master this look, you'll be qualified to be a model, or at least the hostess of *Entertainment Tonight*.

Liposuction

Don't get me wrong. I'm not advising that anyone actually get liposuction. It's just that it is a way of getting rid of some unwanted fat, so I feel I must mention it in this book. Some of you may believe that liposuction is an extreme way of taking off pounds, while others, especially those who live in LA and NYC, think it's as acceptable as paying eight bucks for a cappuccino.

Although liposuction can make you appear thinner, it really isn't an alternative to dieting. Instead, it's a way of getting rid of the stubborn fat that you just can't seem to get rid of no matter how much dieting you do. Some people can do a lifetime of leg lifts or a shootload of sit-ups and still not get rid of their saddlebags or spare tire. It seems that fat can be as stubborn as a pee stain on your new wool rug.

Liposuction is the most common form of cosmetic surgery for both men and women. In fact, the number of yearly procedures is on the rise, increasing 17 percent in 2004 alone. Some of the most common treatment areas for this procedure are the neck, abdomen, chest, and thighs. The best candidates are people who are healthy, fit, at a normal weight, and have skin as taut as Lance Armstrong's heinie.

Liposuction does suck in more ways than one, though. There are complications from the procedure, which vary from asymmetry to lumps and bumps that form from trying to contour the body. There is also a risk of bleeding, excessive bruising, infection, and pockets of fluid that can collect underneath the skin. And, oh yeah, there's the whole death thing to consider as well.

Also, liposuction ain't cheap. Most procedures cost $3,000 to $10,000—many times the price of the food that actually caused the problem in the first place. And sometimes, you'll need more than one treatment. A doctor is limited to removing only five liters of fat at a time (about the size of . . . well, of five one-liter bottles of soda). And finally, liposuction isn't a "lunchtime" procedure, where you're back at the office that same day. In fact, there's about a two-week recovery period, which can eat up all your vacation time as well as your unwanted fat.

So if you have the time, the money, and the desire to risk bleeding, bruising, and death, then go ahead. Who am I to make that kind of decision for you? I have a hard time deciding between paper and plastic.

Gastric Bypass

If you think that liposuction is an extreme way to lose weight, then you'd never go for the option of gastric bypass surgery. Somehow, the idea of being cut open and having your stomach reduced to the size of a tampon may not sit very well with many of you. But if you're more than a hundred pounds overweight and have tried to lose weight on your own, maybe you'd like to know a bit more about the procedure. So I'm here for you, babe. Well, not really here in the true meaning, but here on the printed page and here in spirit and . . . oh, you know what I mean. Let me tell you the real skinny on gastric bypass surgery.

As with liposuction, there are more people having the procedure done today than ever before. Many celebrities have done it, including Al Roker, Carnie Wilson, and Randy Jackson, making stomach stapling a new glamour "Do." Unfortunately, you'll need a celebrity's paycheck to afford the procedure, since the cost of gastric bypass surgery averages between $20,000 and $50,000.

Like liposuction, there are plenty of sucky things about gastric bypass surgery that you should consider before you go under the knife (actually, the term "going under the knife" would be enough of a deterrent for me). Some of the most common side effects of having gastric bypass are:

Nausea and vomiting: These are the most common complications during the first few months after surgery. They're caused by eating too fast, not chewing enough, eating more than your new stomach can hold, or watching really old people kiss.

Dehydration: It's easy to get low on fluids, especially when you're vomiting all day or have diarrhea (another common side effect). Your new stomach can only hold about 3 ounces of fluid at one time, unlike that Big Gulp you were so accustomed to drinking in the past.

Dumping Syndrome: This lovely-sounding medical term occurs when food is passed too quickly from the stomach into the small intestine. "Dumping" can be caused by eating food that's high in sugar, or, of course, by asking your date how many kids he wants when you're only on your first date. But that's a subject covered in my previous book, *Dating Sucks* (yes, I know, it's a shameless plug).

Food Intolerances: After having the surgery, there can be many unexpected food intolerances, especially to red meat, milk, and foods that are high in fiber. This can be a major downer if your favorite food is a beef-and-broccoli milk shake.

Bad Reactions to Overeating: If you overeat after having the surgery, it can lead to vomiting, weight gain, or expansion or even rupture of your new tiny stomach. As you can see, overeating is a lot more serious now than it was before, when about the worst that would happen was that you needed to unzip your pants in order to breathe.

In addition, this surgery carries other risks, including stomach pain, ulcers, gastritis, and threatening calls from your creditors because you're in debt up to your eyeballs after paying for this procedure. And of course, like liposuction, there is always the risk of death.

Self-Acceptance

Besides the solution of getting surgery or wearing higher heels, there is another answer to your weight-loss woes. As long as you've received a clean bill of health from your doctor, maybe you should be more concerned with changing your attitude than your body weight. Maybe the answer is to accept the fact that you may never be a size four like you were in junior high school but then again, you won't get the cystic acne that you had back then either. Maybe you'll never fit into your wedding dress, but then again, you'll never be able to fit back into your sequined sixth-grade culmination skort either, and that never seemed to bother you.

Maybe, just maybe, the lesson to learn from all of this dieting insanity is to accept yourself the way you are. I know that this may seem like more of a struggle than dieting in the first place, but I know for a fact that it can be done. I've known many heavy people over the years who aren't caught up in the whole "skinny" thing. They don't hate themselves when they've polished off two servings of pie or berate themselves for how they look in a bathing suit. Instead, they look at their reflection in the mirror and actually embrace their curves.

I admire women who are able to have such a good mental attitude about their body image. I've tried to do this myself on many occasions, and to some degree, I have achieved it. I accept that no one will ever mistake me for Cindy Crawford. I accept that I will never look good in hot pants. And I accept that I will never again weigh what I did when I got my first driver's license. I also take delight in the fact that I have low cholesterol, a strong heart, and can climb a flight of stairs without breathing too hard, unless of course I'm daydreaming about Matthew Broderick while I'm doing it (maybe it's just me, but I think he's a cutie-patutie).

As long as you eat a fairly healthy diet, get regular check-ups, and do some form of exercise as often as you can, try not to be so hard on yourself. Think of your extra baggage as just one more thing about your body that may not be perfect. Maybe one of your breasts is larger than the other, or you have hair growing on your upper lip. Or maybe you have a cluster of moles on your knee that looks a great deal like the NBC Peacock. *The trick to happiness is to accept your flaws and realize that there are many things in life that are far worse than unwanted cellulite.*

So, embrace your flaws from your double chin to your third nipple (well, maybe not a third nipple, because that's just plain gross). After all your years of dieting struggle, the finest outcome that you can achieve isn't to look good in bike shorts, but instead, to take delight in every nook and cranny and twist and turn that your beautiful body holds. Believe me, if you just accept yourself the way you are, you'll feel more content and happy about yourself than you would from any diet in the world. And this just may be the happy ending that both you and I are both looking for!

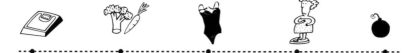

epilogue

Now that I've reached the end of the book, I've also reached the end of my diet. As you may remember from the introduction, I had gained 11 pounds over the previous year, and I was determined to lose it while I wrote this book. You'd think that feat would be quite easy considering it took me six months to write this book (I know that seems long, but sometimes I don't even finish reading a book in that time frame). But unfortunately, I have failed.

When I first started out, I decided to join Weight Watchers. I sat in my meetings and ate my two-point caramel bars despite the fact that they contained Splenda, which gave me so much gas that I now need to repaint the den. After one month, I was down five pounds, which may sound like a lot to some of you, but I was not pleased. I was hoping for a much more substantial weight loss, so I retaliated by eating my weight in doughnut holes.

Next, I tried to forget about eating less food, and focused instead on doing more exercise. I went for an hour-long hike four days a week, and a run around the neighborhood the other three. Unfortunately, the only thing that I ended up losing was the soles on the bottoms of my sneakers. The experience taught me two things, though. One, that I must combine both diet and exercise, and two, that I should never again purchase shoes from a store that contains the word "Bargain" in its name.

I put my diet on hold for a bit while I regrouped, but came back strong weeks later when I tried Atkins yet again. I've had success on that diet in the past, but for some reason, I only lasted on it for three days this time. I'm not much of a meat eater in general, and no amount of hot dogs ever seemed to satisfy my cravings. So that diet ended in one blissful meal of mashed potatoes, pasta, and a can of Almond Roca.

So here it is, six months and several diets later, and after all my hard work, I have only lost 4 pounds. And had it not been for last week's bout with the stomach flu, I probably wouldn't have even lost that much. So here I sit on my slightly smaller behind with 7 more pounds to go, and I wonder if I should accept the fact that I'll never fit into the clothes I bought years back at a wardrobe sale from *A Different World*, or once again go through the hell of yet another diet. Deep down, I know the answer. I know that one path will lead me to contentment while the other path will lead me to a lifetime of frustration and denial. I'll really need to ponder this one for a while. But in the meantime, I hear the sound of last night's lasagna calling my name!

appendix

dieting resources

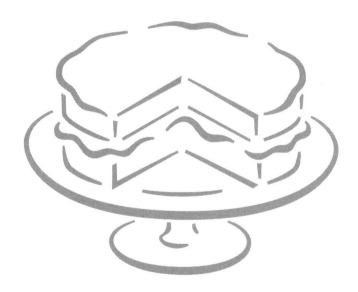

More Information about the
Diets Mentioned in This Book

Weight Watchers: *www.weightwatchers.com*

Jenny Craig: *www.jennycraig.com* or call (800) 597-JENNY

Sugar Busters! Diet: *www.sugarbusters.com*

South Beach Diet: *www.southbeachdiet.com*

Somersizing: *Suzanne Somers' Fast and Easy* by Suzanne Somers (New York: Crown Publishers, 2002); *www.suzannesomers .com*

Ediets: *www.ediets.com*

Cabbage Soup Diet: *www.cabbage-soup-diet.com*

NutriSystem: *www.nutrisystem.com* or call (800) 321-THIN

Popular Workout Tapes

Aerobics: *Carmen Electra's Aerobic Striptease Collection* (also *Carmen Electra's Fit to Strip*)

8 Minute Workouts (Arms/Abs/Buns/Legs)

Weight Training: *Kathy Smith—Timesaver Lift Weights to Lose Weight, Vols. 1 and 2*

Yoga:*A.M. and P.M. Yoga for Beginners*

Pilates: *Classic Pilates Techniques—The Complete Mat Workout Series*

Prenatal Yoga: *Prenatal Yoga with Shiva Rea*

Kickboxing: *Leslie Sansone Walk Away the Pounds—Walk and Kick*

Tai Chi: *Scott Cole's Discover Tai Chi for Beginners—Workout Essentials*

Slow Cooker Cookbooks

Biggest Book of Slow Cooker Recipes (Des Moines, IA: Better Homes and Gardens Books, 2002).

Betty Crocker's Slow Cooker Cookbook (Hoboken, NJ: Betty Crocker, 1999).

The Everyday Low-Carb Slow Cooker Cookbook: Over 120 Delicious Low-Carb Recipes that Cook Themselves, by Kitty Broihier and Kimberly Mayone (New York: Marlowe & Company, 2004).

One Pot Wonders, by Brook Noel (Milwaukee, WI: Champion Press, 2002).

How to Make Love and Dinner at the Same Time: 200 Slow-Cooker Recipes to Heat up the Bedroom Instead of the Kitchen, by Rebecca Field Jager (Avon, MA: Adams Media, 2004).

Great Undergarments
to Hide Trouble Zones

- Lipo in a Box has a full range of slimming undergarments that reduce any trouble zone. To order, go to *www.lipoinabox.com.*
- For an undefined waist, try Waist Nipper from Flexees Underwonder.
- If you have a roll in your belly, try a unitard by Bodyslimmers by Nancy Ganz. It's a bra on top and bicycle-styled shorts on the bottom that make your tummy stay put.
- If you want to make your bust look smaller, try Wacoal Slimline Minimizer bra.
- If you want to make everything look smaller, go to *www.seamlessbody.com.* They have body-shaping garments that lift and shape and tuck everything nicely back into the place where it belongs.

glossary of copyrighted names

7-Eleven	Registered Service Mark of 7-Eleven, Inc.
Ab Lounge	Registered Trademark of Fitness Quest, Inc.
Abba-Zaba bars	Registered Trademark of the Annabelle Candy Co, Inc.
Alpo	Registered Trademark of Alpo Petfoods, Inc.
Amazon	Registered Service Mark of Amazon.com, Inc.
Applebee's	Registered Service Mark of Applebee's International, Inc.
Atkins Diet®	Registered Trademark of Atkins Nutritionals, Inc.
Ball Park frank	Registered Trademark of Hygrade Food Products Corporation
Bally	Registered Trademark of Bally Total Fitness Holding Corporation
Baskin-Robbins	Registered Service Mark of Baskin-Robbins Inc.
Beano	Registered Trademark of Block Drug Company, Inc.
Beef & Broccoli Lean Cuisine	Registered Trademark of Societe des Produits Nestle S.A. Corporation
Ben & Jerry's Phish Food Ice Cream	Registered Trademark of Ben & Jerry's Homemade Holdings, Inc.
Big Gulp	Registered Trademark of The Southland Corporation
Biggest Loser, The	Registered Service Mark of 25/7 productions, LLC, LTD

Blizzard	Registered Trademark of American Dairy Queen Corporation
Bloomin' Onion from Outback Steakhouse	Registered Service Mark of Outback Steakhouse of Florida, Inc.
Bloomingdale's	Registered Trademark of Federated Department Stores, Inc.
Blue's Clues	Registered Service Mark of Viacom International, Inc.
Body by Jake	Registered Trademark of Body by Jake, Inc.
BOTOX	Registered Trademark of Allergan, Inc.
Bowflex	Registered Trademark of Bow-Flex of America, Inc.
Brady Bunch, The	Registered Trademark of Paramount Pictures Corporation
Bridget Jones's Diary	Registered Trademark of Helen Fielding
Bugles	Registered Trademark of General Mills, Inc.
Burger King	Registered Service Mark of Burger King Brands, Inc.
Burger World	Registered Service Mark of Gabriel Gavriel and Politis Spiros
Butterfinger	Registered Trademark of The Curtiss Candy Company
Cabbage Patch Kids	Registered Trademark of Original Appalachian Artworks, Inc.
Cabbage Soup Diet	Abandoned Trademark of The Cabbage Soup Diet Company Ltd.
Campbell's soup	Registered Trademark of CSC Brands LP
Carefree (gum)	Registered Trademark of Nabisco Brands Company
Cheerios	Registered Trademark of General Mills, Inc.
Cheetos	Registered Trademark of Frito-Lay North America, Inc.

Cheez Doodles	Registered Trademark of King Kone Corporation
Cheez Whiz	Registered Trademark of Kraft General Foods, Inc.
Chex cereal	Registered Trademark of Gardetto's Bakery, Inc.
Chex Party Mix	Registered Trademark of Gardetto's Bakery, Inc.
Chili's Guiltess Grill	Registered Trademark of Brinker Restaurant Corporation
Cin-A-Yum pretzel	Registered Trademark of Wetzel's Pretzels LLC LTD
Cinnabon	Registered Service Mark of Restaurants Unlimited, Inc.
Cirque du Soleil	Registered Service Mark of The Dream Merchant Company KFT
Club Med	Registered Service Mark of Club Mediterranee Corporation
Colonel Sanders	Registered Service Mark of Kentucky Fried Chicken Corporation
Cool Ranch Doritos	Registered Trademark of Frito-Lay North America, Inc.
Cool Whip	Registered Trademark of General Foods Corporation
CornNuts	Registered Trademark of Kraft Foods Holdings, Inc.
Crock-Pot	Registered Trademark of Rival Manufacturing Company Corp.
Curves	Registered Service Mark of Curves International, Inc.
Dairy Queen	Registered Trademark of American Dairy Queen Corporation
Del Taco	Registered Service Mark of Del Taco, Inc.

Designing Women	Registered Service Mark of CPT Holdings, Inc.
Diet Coke	Registered Trademark of The Coca-Cola Company Corporation
Ding Dongs	Registered Trademark of Interstate Brands West Corporation
Discman	Registered Trademark of Sony Corporation of America
Ditto jeans	Registered Trademark of Ditto Apparel of California, Inc.
Dodge Caravan	Registered Trademark of Chrysler Corporation
Dolly Madison	Registered Trademark of Interstate Brands Corporation
Double Stuf Oreo cookies	Registered Trademark of Nabisco, Inc.
Dove soap	Registered Trademark of Chesebrough-Pond's Inc.
Dow Jones Averages	Registered Trademark of Dow Jones & Company, Inc.
Eat Right 4 Your Type® diet	Registered Trademark of Peter James D'Adamo
eBay	Registered Service Mark of Kenneth J. Ritter Jr.
eDiets.com	Registered Service Mark of eDiets.com, Inc.
Egg McMuffin	Registered Trademark of McDonald's Corporation
Enron	Registered Service Mark of Enron Corporation
Entenmann's	Registered Trademark of Entenmann's Products, Inc.
Entertainment Tonight	Registered Service Mark of Paramount Pictures Corporation
ER	Registered Service Mark of Time Warner Entertainment Company

Extreme Makeover	Registered Service Mark of American Broadcasting Companies, Inc.
Exxon	Registered Trademark of Exxon Corporation
Food Network	Registered Service Mark of Television Food Network, G.P.
Fritos	Registered Trademark of Frito-Lay, Inc.
Fruit Roll-Ups	Registered Trademark of General Mills, Inc.
Fudgsicle	Registered Trademark of Popsicle Industries, Inc.
Funyuns	Registered Trademark of Frito-Lay, Inc.
Gap (the Gap)	Registered Trademark of Gap (Apparel) Inc.
Garanimal collection	Registered Trademark of Garan, Inc.
Gee Your Hair Smells Terrific™	Common Law Trademark of CGE Enterprises, LLC
Girl Scout Cookies; Thin Mints	Registered Trademark of Girl Scouts of the United States of America Corporation
Goldfish crackers	Registered Trademark of PF Brands, Inc.
Gumby	Registered Trademark of Prema Toy Co., Inc.
Hamburger Helper	Registered Trademark of General Mills, Inc.
Harlequin Romance Enterprises Limited	Registered Trademark of Harlequin
Hersheys bar	Registered Trademark of Hershey Chocolate & Confectionery Corporation
Ho Hos West Corporation	Registered Trademark of Interstate Brands
Hostess West Corporation	Registered Trademark of Interstate Brands
Hummer	Registered Trademark of General Motors Corporation
Hungry-Man Dinner	Registered Trademark of Campbell Soup Company Corporation

In-N-Out Burger	Registered Trademark of In-N-Out Burgers Corporation
iPod nano	Registered Trademark of Apple Computer, Inc.
iTunes downloads	Registered Trademark of Apple Computer, Inc.
J.Crew	Registered Service Mark of J. Crew International, Inc.
Jaws of Life	Registered Trademark of Hurst Performance, Inc.
Jenny Craig®	Registered Service Mark of Jenny Craig, Inc.
Jolly Green Giant	Registered Trademark of Green Giant Company Corporation
Juicy Couture tracksuit	Travis Jeans, Inc.
Just Do It (Nike slogan)	Registered Trademark of Nike, Inc.
Kahlúa	Registered Trademark of Jules Berman & Associates, Inc.
Kenmore	Registered Trademark of Sears Brands, LLC LTD
KFC; Popcorn Chicken	Registered Trademark of Kentucky Fried Chicken Corporation
Kit Kat bar	Registered Trademark of Rowntree Mackintosh Confectionery LTD
Krispy Kreme Doughnuts	Registered Service Mark of Krispy Kreme Doughnut Corp.
Lane Bryant	Registered Trademark of Lane Bryant Purchasing Corp.
Lay's potato chips	Registered Trademark of Frito-Lay, Inc.
La-Z-Boy recliners	Registered Trademark of La-Z-Boy Chair Company Corp.
Lean Cuisine	Registered Trademark of Societe des Produits Nestle S.A. Corporation

Listerine Breath Strip	Registered Trademark of Warner-Lambert Company LLC LTD
Little Debbie	Registered Trademark of McKee Baking Company Corp.
Live with Regis and Kelly	Registered Service Mark of Disney Enterprises, Inc.
Lorna Doone cookies	Registered Trademark of National Biscuit Company Corp.
M&M candy	Registered Trademark of Mars, Incorporated.
Maalox	Registered Trademark of Rhone-Poulenc Rorer Pharmaceuticals, Inc.
Macy's Santa	Registered Service Mark of Federated Department Stores, Inc.
Mallomars	Registered Trademark of National Biscuit Company Corporation
Marie Callender	Registered Trademark of Marie Callender Pie Shops, Inc.
Marshmallow Peeps	Registered Trademark of Just Born, Inc.
Maytag cheese wedge	Registered Trademark of Maytag Corporation
McDonald's	Registered Service Mark of McDonald's Corporation
McGriddles	Registered Trademark of McDonald's Corporation
Melrose Place	Registered Service Mark of Spelling Television, Inc.
Milano cookies	Registered Trademark of Pepperidge Farm Inc.
Milk Duds	Registered Trademark of D. L. Clark Company
Milky Way	Registered Trademark of Mars, Inc.
Miltown	Registered Trademark of Carter Products, Inc.
Minute Rice	Registered Trademark of Kraft Foods, Inc.

Moon Pie	Registered Trademark of Chattanooga Bakery, Inc.
Motrin	Registered Trademark of Johnson & Johnson Corporation
Mrs. Fields	Registered Trademark of Mrs. Fields' Brand, Inc.
Nabisco's 100 Calorie Packs	Registered Trademark of Nabisco Brands Company
NBC Peacock	Registered Service Mark of NBC Universal, Inc.
No-Pest Strip	Common Law Trademark of Hot Shot
Novocain	Registered Trademark of H. A. Metz Laboratories, Inc.
NutriSystem®	Registered Trademark of Nutri/System IPHC, Inc.
Nutter Butter Bars	Registered Trademark of National Biscuit Company Corp.
Old Navy	Registered Trademark of Old Navy (Apparel) Inc.
Oreo Cookies; Oreo Crisps	Registered Trademark of Nabisco, Inc.
Oscar	Registered Trademark of Academy of Motion Picture Arts and Sciences
Outback Steakhouse	Registered Service Mark of Outback Steakhouse of Florida, Inc.
Overeaters Anonymous	Registered Service Mark of Overeaters Anonymous, Inc.
PAM	Registered Trademark of Gibraltar Industries, Inc.
People magazine	Registered Trademark of Time, Inc.
Phen-Fen	Common Law Trademark of David C. Medway

Pillsbury Doughboy	Registered Trademark of The Pillsbury Company Corporation
Pink's	Registered Trademark of Pink's Hot Dogs, Inc.
Polly Pocket	Registered Trademark of Origin Products LTD
Pop Secret; 100 Calorie Pop	Registered Trademark of General Mills, Inc.
Popsicle	Registered Trademark of Lipton Investments, Inc.
Pringles	Registered Trademark of Procter & Gamble Company
Quarter Pounder	Registered Trademark of McDonald's Corporation
Ramen noodles	Registered Trademark of Nissin Foods (USA) Co., Inc.
red Swedish Fish	Registered Trademark of Leaf Sverige AB Joint Stock Co. Sweden
Red Vines	Registered Trademark of American Licorice Company Corp.
Reese's Pieces	Registered Trademark of Hershey Foods Corporation
Rogaine	Registered Trademark of The Upjohn Company Corp.
Ronald McDonald	Registered Service Mark of McDonald's Corporation
Sara Lee	Registered Trademark of Kitchens of Sara Lee, Inc.
Sara's Secrets	Registered Trademark of Television Food Network, G.P.
Sensurround	Registered Trademark of XFRM Incorporated
Seven jeans	Registered Trademark of L'Koral, Inc.

Shabby Chic	Registered Trademark of Shabby Chic, Inc.
Silpat	Registered Trademark of Ets Guy Demarle Joint Stock Co.
Slim-Fast	Registered Trademark of Lipton Investments Inc.
Smart Ones prepackaged foods (Weight Watchers)	Registered Trademark of Weight Watcher's International, Inc.
SnackWell's	Registered Trademark of Kraft Foods Holdings, Inc.
Sno-Caps	Registered Trademark of Ward-Johnston, Inc.
Somersize	Registered Trademark of Port Carling Corporation
Somersizing	Common Law Trademark of Suzanne Somers
Sopranos, The	Registered Service Mark of Time Warner Entertainment Company
South Beach Diet®	Registered Trademark of SBD Trademark Limited Partnership
Spackle	Registered Trademark of Muralo Company, Inc.
Spagos	Registered Service Mark of TSL, LLC, LTD
SPAM	Registered Trademark of Geo. A. Hormel & Company Corp.
Speedo	Registered Service Mark of Speedo International B.V. Corp.
Spider-Man	Registered Trademark of Cadence Industries Corporation
Splenda®	Registered Trademark of McNeil Nutritionals, LLC
Sub-Zero	Registered Trademark of Sub-Zero Freezer Company, Inc.
Sugar Busters! Diet	Registered Trademark of Sugar Busters, LLC
Suzanne Somers ThighMaster	Registered Trademark of Port Carling Corporation

Suzy-Q's®	Registered Trademark of Interstate Bakeries Corporation
Taco Bell; Gordita Supreme	Registered Trademark of Taco Bell Corp.
Target	Registered Service Mark of Target Brands, Inc.
Tastykake	Registered Trademark of Tastykake Investment Company Corp.
Tater Tots	Registered Trademark of Ore-Ida Potato Products, Inc.
Teflon	Registered Trademark of E.I. DuPont De Nemours and Company Corp.
TGI Friday's	Registered Service Mark of TGI Friday's, Inc.
The Limited	Registered Trademark of Limco, Inc.
The Olive Garden	Registered Service Mark of General Mills Restaurant Group, Inc.
TiVo	Registered Service Mark of Tivo, Inc.
Today show	Registered Service Mark of the National Broadcasting Company
Tickle Me Elmo	Registered Trademark of Sesame Workshop Corporation
TrimSpa	Registered Trademark of Nutramerica Corporation
Tums	Registered Trademark of SmithKline Beecham Corporation
Tupperware	Registered Trademark of Dart Industries, Inc.
Twinkies	Registered Trademark of Continental Baking Company
Two and a Half Men	Registered Service Mark of Warner Bros. Entertainment Inc.
Tylenol	Registered Trademark of Tylenol Company
UGG	Registered Trademark of Deckers Outdoor Corporation
Valium	Registered Trademark of Roche Products, Inc.

VIACTIV Chocolate Calcium Chew	Registered Trademark of McNeil Nutrionals, LLC
Viagra	Registered Trademark of Pfizer, Inc.
View, The	Registered Service Mark of American Broadcasting Companies, Inc.
Walkman	Registered Trademark of Sony Kabushiki Kaisha TA Sony Corporation
Wallabees	Registered Trademark of Clarks Wallabies Limited Corporation
WD-40	Registered Trademark of WD-40 Manufacturing Company
Weighing In	Registered Trademark of Television Food Network, G.P.
Weight Watchers	Registered Trademark of Weight Watchers International, Inc.
Wendy's	Registered Trademark of Markdel, Inc.
Wesson Oil	Registered Trademark of Hunt Wesson. Inc.
Wetzel's Pretzels	Registered Service Mark of Wetzel's Pretzels LLC
Whac-a-Mole	Registered Trademark of Bob's Space Racers Inc.
What's Happening!!	Abandoned Service Mark of Columbia Pictures Industries, Inc.
White Castle	Registered Service Mark of White Castle Management Co.
Whopper	Registered trademark of Burger King Corporation
Williams-Sonoma	Registered Trademark of Williams-Sonoma, Inc.
Wonder bread	Registered Trademark of Continental Baking Company Corp.
Zone Diet	Common Law Trademark of Dr. Sears

Index

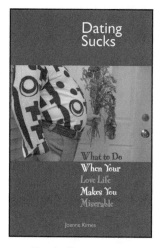
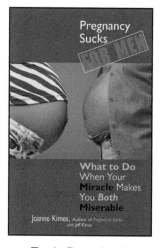
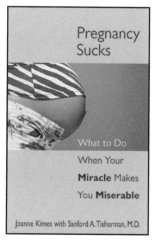

about the author

Joanne Kimes is the coauthor of the bestsellers *Pregnancy Sucks* and *Pregnancy Sucks for Men*. She has written for a number of children's and comedy television shows and has more than two decades of dieting under her belt.